"Dr. Robert A. Nagourney—Nobel-quality researcher and clinical oncologist, extraordinary physician, and creative maverick—is the doctor I'd go to if I had cancer. For decades, with relentless patience, he's been proving that many supposedly incurable cancers can be killed, with greatly reduced harm to the patient, simply by using agents preselected in the laboratory to kill those specific cancer cells. His explanation of why this works, and why it's still misunderstood by many physicians, is a triumph of fact and logic over sloppy assumptions and obsolete habits. Everyone who deals with cancer should read this story, marvel at the results, scrutinize the evidence, and help make the change."

—AMORY B. LOVINS, CHAIRMAN AND CHIEF SCIENTIST,
ROCKY MOUNTAIN INSTITUTE

"In *Outliving Cancer*, Dr. Robert Nagourney brilliantly presents a riveting story of a functional laboratory test that determines the most effective chemotherapy treatment for an individual patient. Everyone's cancer is different. This chemosensitivity assay determines what will work in you, not in the average person. This book is a must-read for any physician involved in the diagnosis and/or treatment of cancer and for cancer patients and their family members seeking the most effective therapy. Functional laboratory testing rescued my wife from the certain death. Her survival, now almost fourteen years later, was entirely due to Dr. Nagourney's identification of a drug combination rarely used in ovarian cancer in 1999, and not recommended by any of the seven gynecologic oncologists she consulted. If you have cancer, this book may save your life!"

—THOMAS PANKE, MD, PRESIDENT, SOUTHERN OHIO PATHOLOGY
CONSULTANTS, INC.; AUTHOR, *PATHOLOGY OF THERMAL INJURY*

"*Outliving Cancer* provides rare insight into the world of a practicing oncologist who is also an innovative research scientist. I highly recommend it to anyone who wants to know why the official war on cancer has progressed so slowly and how it could be made more effective and humane. Dr. Robert Nagourney is a national treasure and in a sane society would be director of the National Cancer Institute."

—RALPH W. MOSS, PHD,
AUTHOR, *CUSTOMIZED CANCER TREATMENT*

"My passion and work for many decades has been in cancer prevention. So it is with great interest that I read Dr. Nagourney's book, *Outliving Cancer.* I can see two major advances changing cancer chemotherapy in the next decade: First, we will have personalized testing with individual tumors. Dr. Nagourney is a pioneer in this area, and he tells an interesting story about how he got there and his successes. Second, chemotherapy drugs that only kill tumor cells and have minimal side effects are coming along rapidly. I also see greater understanding and major advances in preventing cancer. Eating a varied diet so that you get your approximately thirty required vitamins and minerals (and, if you are a smoker, giving up smoking) would be a good start on this. In the meantime, we all are grateful to Dr. Nagourney and the other innovators in cancer chemotherapy and cancer prevention."

—BRUCE N. AMES, PHD, SENIOR SCIENTIST, CHILDREN'S HOSPITAL
OAKLAND RESEARCH INSTITUTE (CHORI)

"Dr. Nagourney has earned international recognition as the most prominent leader in the field of chemosensitivity testing. A more primitive *proliferative* assay led many to reject such testing early on. However, Dr. Nagourney's pioneering work, based on a highly predictive *apoptotic* assay, has benefitted innumerable cancer patients and played a pivotal role in their treatment outcomes. I believe all patients deserve the quality of information that Dr. Nagourney's assay provides, and that in the future, oncology practices will routinely incorporate such testing into the optimal care of patients. I encourage everyone concerned with the treatment of cancer to read *Outliving Cancer.*"

—KEITH I. BLOCK, MD, MEDICAL DIRECTOR, BLOCK CENTER
FOR INTEGRATIVE CANCER TREATMENT; EDITOR-IN-CHIEF,
INTEGRATIVE CANCER THERAPIES, SAGE SCIENCE PRESS;
SCIENTIFIC DIRECTOR, INSTITUTE FOR INTEGRATIVE CANCER
RESEARCH & EDUCATION; AUTHOR, *LIFE OVER CANCER*

"This diary of an oncology physician-scientist is both educational and enjoyable reading for all those interested in cancer and its treatment."

—PHILIP J. DI SAIA, MD, THE DOROTHY MARSH CHAIR
IN REPRODUCTIVE BIOLOGY; PROFESSOR, DEPARTMENT OF
OBSTETRICS AND GYNECOLOGY, UNIVERSITY OF CALIFORNIA,
IRVINE MEDICAL CENTER

Outliving
Cancer

*The Better, Smarter Way
to Treat Your Cancer*

R. A. Nagourney, MD

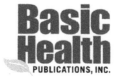

Basic
Health
PUBLICATIONS, INC.

The information contained in this book is based upon the research and personal and professional experiences of the author. It is not intended as a substitute for consulting with your physician or other healthcare provider. Any attempt to diagnose and treat an illness should be done under the direction of a healthcare professional. The publisher does not advocate the use of any particular healthcare protocol but believes the information in this book should be available to the public. The publisher and author are not responsible for any adverse effects or consequences resulting from the use of the suggestions, preparations, or procedures discussed in this book.

Should the reader have any questions concerning the appropriateness of any procedures or preparation mentioned, the author and the publisher strongly suggest consulting a professional healthcare advisor.

Basic Health Publications, Inc.
www.basichealthpub.com

Library of Congress Cataloging-in-Publication Data

Nagournery, Robert A.
   Outliving cancer / Robert A. Nagourney, MD.
      pages cm
   Includes bibliographical references and index.
      ISBN 978-1-59120-306-3 (Pbk.)
      ISBN 978-1-68162-764-9 (Hardcover)

   1. Cancer. 2. Oncology. I. Title.
      RC261.N25 2012
      616.99'4—dc23

                                                      2012045669

Editor: Carol Killman Rosenberg • www.carolkillmanrosenberg.com
Typesetting/Book design: Gary A. Rosenberg • www.thebookcouple.com
Cover design: Dann Froehlich Design

Contents

Acknowledgments, ix

Foreword by Keith I. Block, MD, xiii

Preface, xvii

Introduction, 1

1. A Walk in the Park, 5

2. A Brief History of Chemotherapy and Chemosensitivity Testing, 9

3. Early Scientific Discoveries, 15

4. Anything That Works, 27

5. The Neutrino, 35

6. Epiphany, 39

7. Cell Death Allows for Life, 43

8. Unraveling the Mystery, 47

9. Finally, Rational Therapy, 51

10. Never Give Cancer an Even Break, 57

11. Outliving Hospice, 61

12. East Meets West, 67

13. Garlic, Wine, Chocolate, and More, 73

14. Treatable Cancers Should Be Treated Correctly, 79

15. When All Else Fails, 89

16. The Progress in Treating Kidney Cancer, 103

17. Ah, the Simple Life, 109

18. What to Do When Your Genes Don't Fit, 113

19. Genetic Versus Functional Analysis, 129

20. Targeted Therapies, 135

21. The Future of Cancer Research Lies Behind Us, 147

22. The Causes of Cancer, 151

23. To Cancer and Beyond, 157

APPENDICES

A. Cancer Research Explained, 165

B. What to Expect When You're Expecting a Conversation with Your Oncologist, 169

C. A Practical Guide for the Use of Chemosensitivity Testing, 175

D. Assay Criteria, 185

E. Physician/Patient Advocate Resources, 189

Glossary, 197

References, 219

Index, 223

About the Author, 237

Acknowledgments

I start by thanking Phil Schein, MD, who took me under his wing and guided me through my first experiences with peer-reviewed publications in oncology.

I would also like to thank Larry Weisenthal, MD, PhD, for introducing me to the laboratory technology that has influenced every aspect of my work in oncology.

A very special thanks to Dr. Sheldon Hendler for years of collaboration and brilliant scientific discussion.

Gale (Morrie) Granger for productive collaborations and my introduction to the molecular biology of the human immune system. Kenneth Tew, PhD, who provided me laboratory space and technical support during my fellowship, enabling me to begin my first drug sensitivity lab.

Philip Di Saia, MD, for his support and assistance over the years.

I would like to thank the many surgeons who have collaborated with us to provide tissue samples for our analysis, with particular thanks to Drs. Robert Shuman, Kent Azaren, Imad Shbeeb, Tomi Evans, Anton Bilchik, Peter Dottino, Helmut Schellhas, Sean Cao, Philip Boudreaux, Eugene Woltering, Robert Barone, and Paul Sugarbaker.

I thank Drs. Mel Hoshiko, Joanne Rutgers, Gloria Bertucci, Lowell Rogers, Milton Drachenberg, Julio Ibarra, Steven Romansky,

Emanuel Ferro, Joyce King, Lisa Shane, and Savita Ries, as well as all the members of the Long Beach Memorial Medical Center Pathology Department for their expert assistance in processing tissue samples.

Also, my appreciation to my clinical oncology colleagues, Drs. William Lyons, Jonathan Blitzer, Eknath Deo, Nilesh Vora, John Link, Thomas Asciuto, and Steven Lake, as well as my radiation oncology colleagues, Drs. A. M. Nisar Syed, Ajmel A. Puthawala, and Stephen Doggett for their participation and support in our clinical investigations.

I would especially like to thank my laboratory staff, Steven Evans, Paula Bernard, Eric Federico, and all the past members of our group for overseeing the quality of our operations and dedication to our patients. As well as Shari Burt and Robyn LaFrance for their dedication, perseverance, and multiple abilities.

I'd like to thank Marylyn Paulsen, Tonja Smith, and Debbie Fridman for their hard work in our clinical research department and Cathy Kopy for her continued support.

I also want to thank Loretta Stamos, John Stamos, the entire Stamos family, and the dedicated members of the Vanguard Cancer Foundation for helping us to provide our services to those in need.

A special recognition to John Morrison, Michael and Victoria Campbell, Chip Bupp, Marie-Paule Donsimoni, and Anthony Rothchild for their support.

I thank Dietlind Antretter for collaborations and sponsorship of our developmental program.

I would also like to thank Drs. Ralph Moss, Mark Renneker, Keith Block, Thomas Lodi, and Henry Dreher Jr., who steadfastly promoted and defended our work, referred their patients, and collaborated with us to save the lives of numerous patients over the years.

I would like to thank my parents, Alphonse and Barbara, brother Brian, and sister Sarah for everything that families do.

I would like to thank my wife, Maxine, and my sons Alexander and Adam for their love and support before, during, and throughout the preparation of this book.

Finally, I would like to thank every patient I have had the honor of knowing over the years, who has shown such bravery and strength in the face of adversity. Particular thanks go to those patients who kindly allowed us to include their stories in this book.

This book has been a collaboration among myself, Donna Queza, and Carol Beckerman, without whom it would never have come to be. I thank them for their many hours of dedicated effort, editorial expertise, and encouragement. I also thank William Gladstone of Waterside Productions, Inc., and Norman Goldfind of Basic Health Publications, Inc., for believing in this book and shepherding this project through.

Foreword

As an integrative cancer specialist with more than thirty-two years of clinical care experience and having treated over 15,000 cancer patients, I know firsthand that one of the most critical decisions cancer doctors make is determining which chemotherapy regimen is best for a given patient. There are often many options with no clear-cut reason to choose one over another. Occasionally, existing research data may help a doctor lean toward one regimen, but this rarely addresses the individual's unique biology and tumor characteristics.

Dr. Nagourney's groundbreaking work has provided an invaluable tool in the task of selecting optimal chemotherapy regimens for patients. His work offers doctors a method to better select drugs that are more likely to work on an individual patient's cancer, while avoiding unnecessary protocols that may not work as well, and worse, may cause adverse side effects.

Cancer cells are the wily and tough foot soldiers of a disease that starts silently but can disseminate and eventually overwhelm the body. But detached from their surroundings they are powerless and vulnerable. I remember as a medical student carrying petri dishes of cancer cells between laboratories, trying as best I could to keep them from dying. Impressed with the need to transport them carefully, I was astounded by their fragility when separated from the body and their microenvironment. Yet these were the same cells that had killed my uncle, grandfather, and grandmother before I was sixteen. The contrast was instructive. A light bulb went off in my mind as I realized that our bodies have the ability to coddle or combat cancer, depending on the state or condition of this microenvironment.

In *Life Over Cancer,* I lay out a method for testing and profiling a patient's microenvironment and methods for tailoring a program to shift this toward a cancer fighting as opposed to a cancer promoting terrain. When it comes to chemotherapy, Dr. Nagourney has taken even further aim at using this environment to get a more accurate assessment to determine the more optimal protocol.

Dr. Nagourney's recognition of the importance of this microenvironment is a point of distinction of his methodology. His assay, the EVA-PCD® functional profile, is the only method where the potential effectiveness of a drug is evaluated against the cancer cell in the context of its microenvironment—the tumor stroma or matrix, blood vessels, and inflammatory cells. When a tumor sample arrives at the Rational Therapeutics laboratory, it is broken up into "microspheroids," fragments that preserve the tumor along with its surroundings. Dr. Nagourney can then test drugs in a situation closer to real-life biology than most chemosensitivity tests, which separates cancer cells from their environment.

Another unique feature of the assay is that this test is based on programmed cell death. Programmed cell death is one of the major ways that cancer drugs eliminate tumors. Early tests for chemosensitivity determined whether drugs stopped cells from proliferating, or rapidly dividing, which was previously thought to be the main way that chemotherapy drugs treated cancers. These chemosensitivity tests lacked accuracy, leading many doctors to reject the concept of chemosensitivity testing. More recent research shows that stimulating programmed cell death, also known as apoptosis, is actually a more important mechanism. In apoptosis, a cancer cell self-destructs at the end of its natural lifespan or after experiencing some type of damage. The EVA-PCD assay determines which drugs best activate apoptosis and actually kill tumor cells, rather than just slow the rate at which they multiply.

Dr. Nagourney's laboratory also overcomes a limitation of several other current chemosensitivity tests, which can be described as genomic or biomarker tests. These tests are based on correlating genetic markers or mutations found in tumors with the drugs that are typically found effective in patients with these markers. These markers, which include HER-2, BRAF, KRAS, and others, are definitely important for treatment decisions. The problem is that a single tumor may have multiple markers, some known and some that we have yet to recognize. Because the assay actually applies multiple drugs to each patient's tumor sample, this accounts for the effect of all the markers in the tumor simultaneously.

The potential for improving patients' outcomes using this technique is powerfully demonstrated in Dr. Nagourney's October 2012 publication in the journal *Anticancer Research*. This study tested tumors from thirty-one lung cancer patients at the Rational Therapeutics laboratory. The patients then received the chemotherapy regimens indicated by the functional profile revealed through the assay results. Instead of only a 20 to 30 percent response rate usually seen in lung cancer treatment, nearly 65 percent of these patients had tumor shrinkage or stability. Instead of a typical 9–11 month survival, the average survival of this group was 21.3 months.

This is consistent with what I have experienced with patients using the assay for many years. Some patients have come to us after several regimens of chemotherapy had proven ineffective and they were given no other treatment options. Along with implementing our comprehensive integrative treatment program and chronomodulating chemotherapy—providing drugs in a time-sensitive manner to diminish toxicity while improving response—the findings of the assay provided a direction for treatment that ultimately led to a favorable response.

All cancer patients deserve a comprehensive, individualized, and

integrative approach to care. This approach should include therapeutic nutrition; a personalized bio-behavioral, physical care, and
fitness program; an individualized nutritional supplement regimen
tailored to each patient's unique disease characteristics; biochemical and molecular profiling; and tailoring for optimal drug regimens. The future of cancer treatment will include making treatment
decisions based on each patient's unique tumor characteristics, and
the EVA-PCD assay shows us the way to that future.

The results speak for themselves. If cancer affects you or a loved
one, you owe it to yourself to read the fascinating story recounted
in *Outliving Cancer*. As chemosensitivity testing moves onto center
stage—and mark my words it will—Dr. Nagourney and his functional profile will be revered. For many, this book will be a game-
changer, or perhaps more aptly, a life-changer! This innovative
testing method has helped many of my patients, and it may just provide a genuine solution for you. Please join Dr. Nagourney as he
retraces the challenging development of his methodology, and the
fruits of his work as seen through the outstanding results experienced by those cancer patients who have used his analyses.

Keith I. Block, MD
Medical Director, Block Center for Integrative Cancer Treatment
Editor-In-Chief, *Integrative Cancer Therapies*, Sage Science Press
Scientific Director, Institute for Integrative Cancer Research
& Education
Author, *Life Over Cancer* (Bantam Hardcover)

Preface

As a medical oncology fellow at Georgetown University in the 1980s, I had occasion to attend monthly dinner meetings with guest lecturers from the National Cancer Institute. One evening, Dr. Steven Rosenberg, chief of the surgical branch, came to discuss the management of soft tissue sarcoma. Topics of discussion ranged from the disparities in diagnostic conclusions when pathologists reviewed slides from soft tissue sarcomas (even disagreeing with themselves 25 percent of the time on serial reviews), to the operative management of pulmonary metastases.

What I remember most vividly was Dr. Rosenberg's description of a young man whose soft tissue sarcoma had recurred multiple times in his lungs. Unwilling to yield, Dr. Rosenberg performed more than a dozen separate thoracotomies (surgical explorations of the lung), cherry-picking lesions each time they appeared. That is, until they stopped appearing.

What Dr. Rosenberg had accomplished surgically was what I decided, then and there, would be my medical raison d'etre. I would labor to someday do with chemotherapeutics what Dr. Rosenberg had done with a scalpel: allow my patients to outlive their cancers. Of course, it would be many years before I had the opportunity to realize this dream, but I never wavered from my goal.

This book describes the scientific rationale for my particular approach to cancer medicine—beginning with an interest in cancer as a disease and my good fortune to work with many accomplished physicians, up to the obstacles I encountered along the way. I also expand upon the profound impact the concept of programmed cell death has had upon my worldview.

The reader will come to understand that cancer is not what it once appeared to be, that its management has often been ill conceived and ill applied. And finally, the reader will see that simple insights have enabled me to demonstrably improve my patients' outcomes. By taking a fresh look at some of medicine's most sacrosanct dictates, I have found better, faster, smarter ways to solve even the most complex problems. To some, my work has seemed disruptive, but in an era when oncologic advances are measured with micrometers, I accept the moniker of "disruptor" as a badge of honor.

—Robert A. Nagourney, MD

Introduction

The parable of the tortoise and the hare, attributed to Aesop, tells of the cocky hare who taunts the lumbering tortoise. The tortoise then challenges the hare to a race. The faster hare, far in the lead, stops for a nap and allows the tortoise to pass him. Author Thomas Henry Croxall in his interpretation coined the phrase "The more haste, the worse speed," to describe the unexpected outcome. But is it unexpected? Are we not all witness to headstrong individuals, so convinced of the merit of their approach to problems that they'll risk all in pursuit of their purported goal? Are not the dot.com and more recent real estate bubbles reflections of this mindset? More to the point, are not those who lose the most in these scenarios the unwitting participants, and not the purveyors of these ill-conceived schemes?

Cell theory, developed by Theodor Schwann and Matthias Jakob Schleiden and articulated by Rudolf Virchow in 1839, defined three fundamental principles of life. First, all living organisms are composed of cells. Second, the cell is the smallest unit that comprises all of the features that define a living creature. Finally, all life is predicated upon cell division. It is the last point more than any other that launched the modern concept of cancer.

Malignant cells, it was reasoned, grew more, because these cells divided more. The "hare" of cancer could outpace its slower, benign "tortoise" counterpart by winning the battle of the birthrate. The first chemotherapy drugs, nitrogen mustard and shortly thereafter aminopterin, were examples of therapy predicated upon the deeply held belief that cancer was running faster. With the increasingly broad application of these drugs and their chemical derivatives during the 1950s and 1960s, the allure of chemotherapeutics slowly paled, as toxicities overtook response rates and remissions proved brief and unsustainable.

Undaunted, the next generation of oncologists launched the era of combination chemotherapy heralded by alphabet-soup regimens with names like MOPP, m-BACOD, and CHOP. It wasn't that chemotherapy didn't work, they opined, it was that we were not giving it correctly. Non-cross-resistant drugs needed to be given in carefully constructed sequences to capture tumor cells in their most "vulnerable" state, cell division. This mind-set careened along for another decade, culminating in regimens with names like PRO-MACE-CYTABOM that were so toxic and complex that even the treating physicians couldn't understand them.

The 1993 "battle-of-the-bands" that pitted the original four-drug CHOP regimen for lymphoma against its increasingly complex offspring brought the entire field to a standstill, when "old-fashioned" CHOP proved every bit equal in all but one category: it killed fewer patients.

"But where to from here?" was the cry, and "dose escalation" was the response.

"If some is good, more is better" became the guiding principle of investigators who came to be known as bone marrow transplanters. These researchers decided to push the dose envelope right up to the point where patients would die. In fact, many of them did. In order to rescue these patients from certain death, bone marrow elements removed from the patients themselves, or a close relative, were infused into the body to salvage the immune system that these doctors had just succeeded in destroying. Had the process actually worked—that is, had the myriad breast cancer and other solid tumor patients who signed up in droves to participate in these programs actually been helped—then it might have been worth it. But it didn't work, not at all.

Five large studies examined the impact of bone marrow transplantation on survival in breast cancer and only one achieved positive results. And that one, it turned out, was fraudulent. With a resounding thud the most recent version of modern cancer therapeutics had faltered, big time.

In any discipline, it becomes necessary to take stock when expectations aren't being met and seemingly lovely theories collapse under the weight of irrefutable fact. The most productive of these introspective exercises are often the most painful. While the oncologic rank and file turned to navel-gazing, the more insightful investigators went back to the drawing board and raised uncomfortable questions that dealt with the most profound tenets of cancer therapeutics. By throwing off the yoke of a century-long premise that cancer was a disease of overactive cell division, scientists like John Reed, MD, PhD; Carlo Croce, PhD; Robert Horvitz, PhD; and many others challenged the prevailing thinking and forged a new direction in cancer biology.

This book is one interested physician scientist's application of those same principles to cancer therapy. It seems that cancer is not so "incurable" or "untreatable" as we have been taught to believe. Instead, it is driven by processes and principles that escaped the notice of earlier scientists. Like the theories that the Earth was at the center of the solar system or that it was flat, cancer biology must now be viewed in a more modern context if it is to be conquered.

Outliving Cancer is the tale of discovery and enlightenment that enabled me as a physician to rethink what it was that I was doing in my practice, to rethink what cancer was, and finally to develop a new way to treat the disease. The cancer patient, it turns out, is the "tortoise." Their slow and deliberate efforts enable them to ultimately outpace their cancers. Slow and steady, patients maintain the equilibrium of cell dynamics, known as homeostasis, that guides

them to the finish line. When first I pondered the "source docu-
ments" from which some of my thinking arose, I had not imagined
the need to look back 2,500 years, but it may be Aesop's fable
(620–564 BC) that best captures the principles of this book.

1

A Walk in the Park

On Sunday, December 12, 1982, I spent the afternoon in Washington, D.C., at the National Gallery of Art where I sat quietly and pondered the Gainsborough portrait of Mrs. Richard Brinsley Sheridan. It's a wistful painting and has always left me with a sense of melancholy. I drove back to my apartment on Massachusetts Avenue and took a walk in Rock Creek Park, adjacent to my building. Long yellow rays of late afternoon sunlight broke through the barren trees. As the Rock Creek murmured through partially snow-covered stones and tree branches, my sense of melancholy deepened.

It had been almost six months since I arrived in Washington, D.C., serving as a first-year fellow of medical oncology at the Lombardi Cancer Center at Georgetown University. Prior to my arrival, during my residency at the University of California, Irvine, I had prided myself on my medical skills. I could start an IV on any patient, intubate any patient, and aspirate fluid from any body cavity. But now, in the middle of the first year of my oncology fellowship, every single patient under my care died a miserable death.

No one got better, not anyone, ever.

No matter how much I liked the former American Consul General from Montreal (where I had attended medical school) or the twenty-nine-year-old pancreatic cancer victim who improved so dramatically, but equally briefly, from my last-ditch efforts, every single patient died. I had lost my mojo.

My lifelong desire to be a physician, healer, and comforter had been replaced by my role as a tormentor. Patients weren't only dying, I was poisoning them. I hated oncology. I was beginning to hate medicine. Having wanted to be a doctor my whole life, I was beginning to hate my life. It was neither the work schedule (though extreme) nor the penury (also extreme). No, it was the fact that I could no longer practice medicine. Everyone died, and I didn't seem to be able to do anything about it.

Although I had never seriously considered suicide in my life, I began to wonder whether I should really go on living.

As I walked along, with the light dusting of snow crunching below my feet, I had a breakthrough. I realized that however poorly my patients did and however ineffective my treatments might be, *I* didn't do it.

I didn't give anyone cancer; they got it on their own. I didn't cause them to die. They were dying on their own, and I wasn't doing anything to stop it. However dismal my track record, I realized that at least I was on the right side of the battle—I was trying.

It was that epiphany that enabled me to continue my fellowship and complete my two-year training program. If I was guilty, I wasn't guilty of an error of commission. Rather, I was guilty of an error of omission. I wasn't actively killing my patients—I just wasn't actively saving them.

I resolved that the rest of my training, indeed the remainder of my career, would be dedicated to finding better ways to treat this scourge. At the beginning of my second year of fellowship, the opportunity to pursue that goal would present itself.

THE DREAMS OF CHILDHOOD

When you ask a child what they want to do when they grow up, many will say that they want to be a policeman, fireman, astronaut, or president. Some will say they want to be a doctor.

Most never go on to realize these childhood dreams. But not me.

From the age of five I was certain. I knew I would be a doctor, and I planned to go to the Columbia University School of Medicine in New York City. My choice of Columbia came completely from my uncle, the physician, who had studied there. I didn't really know what Columbia was, but I did know that I was absolutely, positively going to be a doctor.

After high school graduation, I attended Boston University as a chemistry major with basic research in biochemistry. When I was a pre-med student there was no shortage of anecdotes from well-meaning friends about the straight-A student with perfect MCAT (Medical College Admission Test) scores who couldn't get into medical school. Unfazed, I never once questioned whether or not I would be a doctor. With my acceptance to several medical schools, I began my studies at Georgetown University, subsequently completing them at McGill University in Montreal (no, not Columbia). What I was less sure about—in fact, utterly unsure about—was what kind of doctor I wanted to be. I was pretty sure I didn't want to be a surgeon. And I was almost equally as sure that I didn't want to be involved in cancer.

FINDING DIRECTION

In the 1970s, cancer and cancer therapy were distinctly unappealing. Few patients improved, but everyone suffered the side effects of chemotherapy. When I found myself as a first-year medical student seeking basic research opportunities, I first visited with a biochemist. With my degree in chemistry, basic research in biochemistry, and a genuine love of organic chemistry, I trained my sights on laboratory work in this field. The first faculty member with whom I met was conducting studies on gastrointestinal absorption. When I realized one of his principal areas of work were the chemical components that make human stool brown, I decided to look elsewhere.

I then met Dr. Mark Smulson in the Department of Biochemistry

at Georgetown University. A clever biochemist, Dr. Smulson looked
a bit like a beatnik and smoked a pipe. He had a gravelly voice,
glassy eyes, and a black, trimmed beard. We talked at length about
my interests and he said, "I know who you should work with—Phil
Schein."

Dr. Philip S. Schein had just arrived at Georgetown from the
National Cancer Institute. He and his group of young investigators
had succeeded in treating Hodgkin disease. They then moved on to
a combination of therapies for the treatment of non-Hodgkin lymphoma. He brought his team to Georgetown and set up shop. Dr.
Schein's entire program had been shoehorned into office spaces
located on the second story of the old Georgetown Medical School.
I walked in and was met by Jackie, his secretary. She was cheerful,
friendly, and ushered me into Phil's tiny office.

Phil was young and energetic—with the look of a tennis cham-
pion about to pounce on the next serve. He asked what I was interested in and I told him biochemistry. He said that his lab was
studying new forms of chemotherapy. They were synthesizing collections of compounds and he was testing them on pancreatic cancer. He showed me a chemical structure and pointed out one of his
newest compounds: "an amide." I examined the structure and then
pointed out that it was in fact "an imide." He peered back at me, a
bit startled, smiled and said, "You're right . . . would you like a job?"
"Okay," I replied.

I was introduced to the laboratory staff and, within weeks, was
conducting my own experiments examining the dose-response relationships of novel compounds both in animals and by chemical reaction. Ironically, my previous aversion to cancer research evaporated
as I suddenly became immersed in that exact field of medicine. As
in any medical specialty, once you've published in a few peer-
reviewed manuscripts there's no turning back. After I completed
medical school and my residency, I found myself back at Georgetown University as a fellow in medical oncology.

2

A Brief History of Chemotherapy and Chemosensitivity Testing

Scientific discovery is often serendipitous. This was certainly the case on the night of December 2, 1943, when German bombers attacked the Italian port city of Bari and sank the U.S. ship *John Harvey*. The U.S. Navy had stockpiled mustard gas onboard, which they intended to use if German forces initiated chemical warfare. This was highly classified information. With the release of the mustard gas from the ship's hull, soldiers, Navy personnel, and innocent bystanders were exposed to the effects of this toxic agent.

As a class of chemicals, the mustards (including both sulfur and nitrogen) had been known since the 1850s. Indeed, investigators observed that poisoning with these substances caused leukopenia (a condition of less than the normal level of white blood cells) and bone marrow aplasia (failure of the bone marrow to produce sufficient numbers of blood cells), as early as 1919 (Krumbhaar 1919). However, it wasn't until the Bari incident that the biological impact of nitrogen mustard upon humans was fully appreciated. The stunning impact of nitrogen mustard exposure upon bone marrow, lymphoid tissue, and the gastrointestinal tract led Louis Goodman, MD, Alfred Gilman, MD, PhD; and Thomas Dougherty, PhD, to formally analyze the effects of these compounds in mice that had been transplanted with a form of cancer known as lymphosarcoma. The successful eradication of cancer in these animals in experiments

9

conducted during the 1940s and 1950s led to human clinical trials a decade later.

While investigators at Yale continued their study of nitrogen mustard, Sydney Farber, MD, and his colleagues in pediatric oncology at Harvard, were closing in on a different but related clue. Recognizing that acute leukemia cells blossomed when exposed to folic acid (a B vitamin known to be critical for the production of genetic material) Dr. Farber created a decoy molecule, aminopterin, which deprived these cells of their precious DNA. Like the original experiences with the mustards for lymphoma, aminopterin proved effective in leukemia, establishing that even the most disseminated forms of cancer could be managed with medicines. The era of cancer chemotherapy was born.

What these two discoveries had in common was the underlying premise that chemotherapy worked by disrupting cellular proliferation and that the cell's DNA was the target of interest. Numerous chemical compounds developed over the next thirty years for the treatment of cancer only perpetuated this thinking. Decades later, these premises would be revisited, but only after millions of patients had received cytotoxic drug combinations of increasing intensity and complexity. Many responded and a few were cured, but absolutely every one of them suffered significant toxicity, and the search for a better way to deliver chemotherapy was upon us.

TESTING INSTEAD OF GUESSING

To a reasonable person, using a test to choose chemotherapeutic drugs before they are prescribed to patients would seem intuitively obvious. Even more so when one considers the profound toxicity and relatively low response rates associated with most cancer therapies. Indeed, clinical investigators have pursued this avenue of research since 1954 (Black 1954).

With each passing decade thereafter, a new methodology would rise and ultimately fall, failing to meet the needs of patients and physicians. Then, a landmark paper was published in the *New England Journal of Medicine* (*NEJM*) in June of 1978 (Salmon 1978). This article described the clonogenic (human tumor stem cell) assay (test). Sidney Salmon and colleagues, borrowing from groundbreaking work conducted by investigators in Toronto, applied the concept of human tumor stem cells to the study of chemosensitivity. Within months of that publication, hundreds, if not thousands, of laboratories all around the world focused their attention on the human tumor stem cell (now often referred to as the Salmon) assay. And the University of Arizona, Tucson—Salmon's university—became the focal point of clonogenic studies. The National Cancer Institute (NCI) established a drug-screening program based on this technique and entrepreneurs launched commercial laboratories offering it as a service.

I remember reading the journal article as a medical student and feeling a sense of excitement. Perhaps the dismal results I was already experiencing, might—for the first time—be meaningfully improved. I knew only too well from the black humor of the fellows (while I was a medical student in an oncology lab) that chemotherapy wasn't working. Regardless of the assay's ultimate validity, the concept was enormously appealing. However, my personal interests in the assay had to wait until I finished medical school and most of my residency. Only then would I meet Dr. Larry Weisenthal.

Dr. Weisenthal had read the same *NEJM* article during his fellowship at the NCI. Like so many other investigators at that time, he became an expert in clonogenic assays. He was also developing a second test, using cell-staining characteristics to measure drug effects that focused on the uptake of colored dyes (staining) that occurs in cells that lose metabolic viability. While taking an elective course as a third-year resident, I spent a few weeks in Dr. Weisenthal's laboratory. He kindly instructed me on both the clonogenic assay and his newly developed differential staining endpoint.

Everything was progressing in the field until 1983 when the *NEJM* published an analysis of more than 6,000 patients and reported that the clonogenic assay was a bust (Selby 1983). By the time that article appeared, I had already recognized the assay's shortcomings and was exploring alternatives. With all the inherent problems of the clonogenic process, the staining assay developed by Dr. Weisenthal seemed so much more appealing. It was my research on the differential staining method that I took with me the following year to Georgetown.

The problem was, the 1983 *NEJM* article had done irreparable damage to the field of chemosensitivity testing and to everyone engaged in the work. We were all tarred with the same brush.

So, why didn't the clonogenic assay work? I remember having that discussion high atop the Hammer Building at, of all places, Columbia University, with Dr. Sol Spiegelman. Dr. Spiegelman, a scientist of immense accomplishments, was intrigued by Dr. Salmon's supposition that cancers propagated through the growth of stem cells and that stem cells needed to be the target of therapeutic intervention. While I didn't disagree with the importance of self-renewing cells (stem cells), it was unclear to me whether capturing any cell during its growth phase would provide the information needed to select chemotherapeutics.

After all, growing cells, like a child in utero, cannot tolerate toxins in their environment. What might be a tolerable treatment for an adult (say, an aspirin) could result in severe birth defects for a child in early gestation.

Similarly, cancer cells that are rapidly dividing are prone to the toxic effects of drugs in ways that artificially sensitize them, thus yielding results of low predictive validity.

In a military context, Sun Tzu, the famed Chinese warrior-philosopher, said, "A military operation involves deception. Even though you are competent, appear to be incompetent. Though effective, appear to be ineffective." When the growing tumor appears incompetent following exposure to drugs and combinations in the test tube, it succeeds in fooling the clinician into believing it will respond in the body. But it is the tumor's more defended (nonproliferating) brethren who will weather the assault of chemotherapeutic drugs and live to fight another day.

What was needed was an ability to measure the resistance of the most defended cells, not the most vulnerable. The clonogenic assay, like all other growth-based assays, could not provide this information.

In retrospect, the failure of the clonogenic assay should have been obvious. The disappointment was that people could not see around that failure to other, more productive solutions. A failing that continues to this day.

3

Early Scientific Discoveries

The first six months of my medical oncology fellowship profoundly undermined my enthusiasm, even my willingness to continue in this field. However, my moment of clarity in Rock Creek Park sparked a new sense of excitement and a desire to re-create the work I had started the previous summer in Dr. Weisenthal's lab.

On July 1, 1983, with my first year of oncology fellowship at the Georgetown Lombardi Cancer Center behind me (the dedicated clinical year), I moved from the clinical center to the research department in the basement of the facility. It was there, under the tutelage of Kenneth Tew, PhD, director of molecular pharmacology, that I was given bench space, material support, and some technical assistance to create a human tumor chemosensitivity laboratory. With my workload reduced from daily clinics and ward rounds to half-day clinics twice a week, I spent weekdays, evenings, and weekends toiling in the lab. I focused initially on blood-borne tumors in the form of leukemias and lymphomas, because of their ready availability (a simple tube of blood), and the ease with which the cells could be isolated (density centrifugation). Over time, I moved to the more difficult study of solid tumors. As opposed to the leukemias, solid tumors demanded skills in microspheroid (cluster) isolation and cell separation.

Those were heady times. Like a kid in a candy shop, I could test anything I wanted. After all, I was testing human cancer cells, but I didn't have to administer the drugs to patients to see if they worked. The results became increasingly interesting. Among my first findings was the observation of synergy between the chemotherapy drug 5-FU and the biological agent alpha-interferon. Synergy, also known as supra-additivity, is that unique event that occurs when two drugs added together provide superior activity over either agent alone. This was subsequently published in a text-book (Woolley 1986).

I then redoubled my efforts in leukemia patients. As previously noted, the cells were easy to isolate and there were many active drugs available. Another early observation regarded the effects of high concentration exposures to the drug ARA-C (arabinofuranosyl cytidine) in patients with acute myelogenous leukemia (AML), the most common form of adult leukemia. What I found was that in the test tube, up to a point, the more ARA-C I exposed the cells to, the more cells I killed. I wondered whether it would be possible to increase the normal dose of ARA-C to achieve the same effect in patients.

Coincidentally, a Baltimore-based research group had just reported the use of high dose ARA-C for the treatment of resistant AML.

As fate would have it, an opportunity to test this hypothesis arose. One of my co-fellows at the Georgetown program was taking a long weekend and asked me to cover his shift on a Thursday night. It so happened I had been invited to an Organization of American States black-tie reception that same evening. But I agreed to cover, hoping for a quiet evening. Around 10 PM, I was paged. The American Consul General from Barbados was arriving at Andrews Air Force Base on a military transport. He was desperately ill with AML and would require immediate admission to the hospital.

The call from the emergency room came later that evening. The patient was quickly processed through the ER, and then seen by the medical intern and resident. He then awaited my arrival. Lacking the time to return home, change, and make it to the hospital, I arrived at the patient's room in a tuxedo. He inquired where in the pecking order I belonged. I explained that he had seen the junior resident, senior resident, and I was now the fellow.

He asked if I always arrived in black tie. I replied, "Of course." He then inquired who came after me. "The attending physician," I replied. "And do they wear tuxedos as well?" "Oh, no," I smiled, "for the attending physicians it's white tie only."

We became fast friends and I quickly began his treatment with the standard 3-plus-7 induction chemotherapy used in all AML patients. Unfortunately, he did not achieve a remission. The bone marrow aspiration confirmed the relapse and yielded ample cells for me to test in the lab. Interestingly, his leukemia cells responded favorably when subjected to higher doses of ARA-C. The opportunity to test the hypothesis was at hand. Few good options were available, but his cells revealed the desired profile and the papers on high dose administration had just been published. The Lombardi Cancer Center at Georgetown University was about to enter the era of high dose ARA-C.

Much to my delight and amazement, the Consul General achieved a complete remission. I compiled his story with that of several other patients into an abstract that was reported at the 1984 American Society of Clinical Oncology meeting in Toronto (Nagourney 1984). The success of that high dose schedule presaged a significant change in leukemia therapy. Researchers around the world developed similar schedules and came to include high dose ARA-C as the so-called "consolidation" therapy for patients in remission. Today, more than 40 percent of AML patients are cured of their disease using this strategy. These results are as good as those associated with the more aggressive bone marrow transplant approaches. While I cannot claim that my work influenced the adoption of this approach, I could see early on, through the lens of my laboratory, the merit of its use.

Attending the meeting in Toronto, I felt reenergized. Maybe I could change the outcomes for my patients. Perhaps medical oncology didn't need to be so grim. With the recent successes that I witnessed, one thing seemed certain: I could never go back to the blind administration of chemotherapeutic drugs again.

AN ETHICAL DILEMMA

In July 1984, I was comfortably ensconced in La Jolla, California, as a hematology fellow at the Scripps Institute. Not only is La Jolla one of the most beautiful places in the world, but I was granted lab space and an opportunity to further study my interest in the tissue culture techniques I had begun at Georgetown. And I had the good fortune of working with Dennis Carson, MD.

A creative thinker and capable scientist, Dr. Carson had overseen the synthesis of a novel compound for the treatment of leukemias. The drug, 2-chlorodeoxyadenosine (2CDA), was specifically designed to mimic a well-recognized immune deficiency caused by the loss of an enzyme—adenosine deaminase. For reasons that were not entirely understood, the loss of adenosine deaminase resulted in depletion of T-lymphocytes. This subset of the immune system, distinct from B-lymphocytes, served as the command post for immune surveillance. The absence of T-cells left the immune system rudderless. Children afflicted with this genetic disease suffered repeated infections, ultimately leading to death. The children with severe combined immunodeficiency (SCID) were known as "bubble children" because they needed to live in a completely enclosed sterile environment for their entire lives. By partially re-creating this condition pharmacologically through the administration of 2CDA, Dr. Carson and his team could cause malignant lymphocytes to die without triggering the full-blown SCID.

Based upon their research using the popular cell-line systems (themselves derived from human T- and B-cell leukemias and lymphomas), these investigators were convinced that 2CDA would be selectively effective for leukemias and lymphomas that arose in the T-cell subpopulations.

When I arrived at the Scripps Clinic, 2CDA was under preliminary investigation for the treatment of T-cell lymphoma. With the kind gift of a small amount of the drug from Dr. Carson, I launched an analysis of this novel compound in human leukemia cells removed directly from the bloodstream of patients. Much to my surprise, I observed significant activity in T-cell, B-cell, and myeloid leukemias. However, I did not observe any activity in the B-cell neoplasm known as multiple myeloma.

After reading a paper describing the use of a related drug, pentostatin, which acted in a manner similar to 2CDA, I obtained cells from the spleen of a patient with a rare cancer—hairy cell leukemia. I was convinced that pentostatin's effect could be duplicated with 2CDA. As I documented in my laboratory notebook, 2CDA was indeed active in this disease. I was elated—I had made a discovery.

I believed that 2CDA would work for patients with hairy cell leukemia. However, when I approached the senior investigators at Scripps suggesting that we test 2CDA in hairy cell, I was met with the same response that I would encounter repeatedly over the ensuing years. Namely, the laboratory model (like the related clonogenic assay) did not provide relevant information for the prediction of clinical response. I was informed that there would be little reason to apply my findings in the form of a clinical trial.

Several years later—after I had left Scripps to join the University of California, Irvine (UCI)—a landmark paper by investigators from the Scripps Clinic established 2CDA as the curative therapy for hairy cell leukemia, a therapy that continues to be used to this day. To my recollection, it did not mention my previous observations.

Despite my disappointment that I was unable to launch the trial to confirm the initial observation, I did generate one more interesting bit of data with that compound: an observation of extraordinary synergy between 2CDA and members of a class of drugs known as alkylating agents, such as Cytoxan. I subsequently reported this and related findings in a paper published in the *British Journal of Cancer* (Nagourney 1993). Interestingly, this too proved to

be a seminal observation. The closely related combination of fludarabine and Cytoxan went on to be the preferred treatment for
chronic lymphocytic leukemia (CLL) and low-grade lymphoma, two
of the most common blood cancers.

At the completion of my fellowship, I was recruited to join the
faculty at UCI. At that point in time, I was certain that the study of
human tumor primary cultures would continue to provide important insights and even more certain that convincing my colleagues
would be an uphill battle.

EARLY DISCOVERIES OF A MORE POLITICAL NATURE

My experience at Scripps taught me that the academic community
functioned as a hierarchy of senior investigators dictating to junior
investigators. The merit of one's observations was subservient to the
position that one held in the hierarchy. Scientific discoveries were
only discoveries when made by the right person at the right institution.

There is an old joke that one of my UCI colleagues told me. It
tells of a breakthrough treatment that resulted in the permanent
elimination of all measurable tumor in every mouse treated. When
the presenter of the paper was asked by an astonished member of
the audience when this brilliant new treatment might receive
approval for the treatment of patients, the presenter responded,
"When the mice are treated at Harvard."

Having completed two fellowships, a residency, and medical
school, I wondered whether I really wanted to continue in this vein.
Over cocktails at an American Society of Clinical Oncology meeting with the senior faculty of several East Coast medical institutions,
I was asked by my former boss Dr. Schein what I was working on.
I told him—tongue in cheek, but not entirely—"my duck jibe." (A
duck jibe is an advanced maneuver conducted by windsurfers when
changing direction under high wind conditions, often in the midst
of wave jumping.) At the time, I had decided to take the summer

off and windsurf every day. I worked the night shift in the Harbor View Hospital emergency room, which left me free to spend my days as I chose, and I chose to windsurf.

It was during this idyllic summer that my colleague Dr. Weisenthal told me of a new, federally funded grant program—the Small Business Innovation Research (SBIR). The grant was designed to sponsor the development of biotech companies. Two phases were provided: Phase I, a pilot study; and Phase II, a definitive study. We decided to apply, and I spent the fall of 1985 completing grant applications.

We succeeded in obtaining one of the two Phase I grants for which we had applied. Now, all we needed to do was create a biotech company.

With some seed funding from Long Beach Memorial Medical Center and the assistance of the lead pathologist Dr. James Baker, we established Oncotech, Inc., and set up shop in a medical building near the hospital. We hired staff and began conducting experiments to prove that human tumors resistant to chemotherapeutics could be resensitized by pre-incubation with calcium channel blockers, glutathione depletors, and protein kinase C inhibitors. We succeeded in completing every requirement of the grant and submitted our Phase II application, expecting glowing reviews.

Unbeknown to us, the grant reviewers who had approved our initial submission were no longer part of the process. Those enlightened investigators, who had read our original application for its merit, were replaced by the same people who had turned down all of our prior papers and grant submissions. Despite meeting every expectation of the grant's outline, our Phase II application was denied.

Luckily, the successful pursuit and receipt of an SBIR grant, even Phase I, resounded across the investment community. Oncotech became a hot topic. We were approached by venture capitalists interested in sponsoring the expansion of our program. As a physician and academic, I knew little of the world of investments, particularly of venture capital. My cofounder and I turned down a generous offer

of $3 million for 51 percent of the business, worried that the control-
ling interest by the venture arm of SmithKline (SR-1) would immediately handcuff us as founders. We opted instead for less money
and less control by investors: $1 million for a 28 percent interest in
the company. For anyone who has participated in the venture capital game, you know only too well how this played out.

First, we needed a larger building. Then, we had to hire a head-
hunter to locate a director of marketing and a CEO. We needed a
lab director, a CFO, and a sales staff. And no sooner did this begin
then we were out of money again. And now came the controlling
interest argument.

"Would you rather have a big piece of a small pie or a small piece
of a big pie?" said Jay Raskin, one of Oncotech's investors, arguing
in favor of our accepting additional money. The alternative was to
close the company. I wish, in retrospect, we would have played a
little more brinksmanship. With the second round of financing came
an entirely new group of deep-pocketed investors and the outcome
was written in stone. The venture capitalists, too timid to support
the scientists, insisted (now that they had controlling interest) that
we recruit a scientist whose expertise lay in the field of tumor cell
proliferation—exactly the opposite of everything the company was
founded to do.

David H. Kern, PhD, was recruited from the Sepulveda Veteran's
Administration to develop and commercialize a growth-based assay
that didn't work, indeed couldn't work, and ultimately resulted in
the collapse and bankruptcy of Oncotech two decades later following its sale to the Danish concern Exiqon in 2008.

This "son-of-clonogenic assay" methodology was marketed
under the name "extreme drug resistance." This was a concept that
I helped develop and originally called HGDR (high grade drug
resistance). It occurred to me, as the medical director of Oncotech
during those unfortunate years, that the assay didn't work, that I
was reporting useless information, and as a medical doctor I could-
n't clearly defend my activities.

Due to the conditions of the assay (designed to seek any level of drug activity as a screening methodology) this ill-conceived cell proliferation assay consistently identified drug activity for inactive drugs in drug-resistant diseases.

Although the assay was conducted carefully and was consistently reproducible, when applied to patients in the clinic it was utterly and totally inaccurate. Vinblastine is not and has never been active in colon cancer, not ever, but Dr. Kern's assay turned up vinblastine activity in virtually every colon sample.

It wasn't a technical issue. That is, the execution of his assay was technically superb. It was just that growing cells, by nature, are very sensitive to chemotherapeutic drugs. And the high concentrations used by Dr. Kern further elevated the artificiality of the results. When proliferating, drug-sensitive cells are exposed to unnaturally high drug concentrations, you get growth inhibition almost all the time. The problem was that as the only practicing oncologist in the company, I knew only too well that colon cancer, lung cancer, and melanoma were not drug sensitive. Certainly not remotely as drug sensitive as Dr. Kern's assay would suggest.

I called a meeting of the company and stated that I was going to close Oncotech. My fiduciary responsibilities were superseded by a solemn oath—the Hippocratic oath. Oncotech's drug sensitivity data was irrelevant and clinically useless. As the only legal laboratory scientist on the premises, I held the trump card—the license that kept the laboratory open. Oncotech was closing.

By now, Oncotech was bristling with staff—a CEO, a CFO, a VP of Marketing, a marketing director, a sales staff, and a host of lab staff. Every job hung in the balance and I was standing my ground. So, as venture capital–backed CEOs are known to do, they organized an offsite retreat.

We met in the morning and reviewed the dilemma. Dr. Kern held that his lab was absolutely precise, that the data was consistent, his quality controls and oversight were beyond reproach. Everything was as it should be. I argued that medical science and laboratory services are not conducted in a vacuum, that Dr. Kern's highly reproducible results were ridiculous and had no bearing on human cancer outcomes. I would never, as long as I lived, sign another report stating that colon cancer was sensitive to vinblastine— NEVER.

LOOKING FOR THE SILVER LINING

Dr. Weisenthal, who in his role straddled the fence between clinic and laboratory, and I examined Dr. Kern's data. One set of results stood out in his analyses. It was the comparison of assay results against clinical outcomes in more than 400 studies. There was one interesting finding. If you examined Dr. Kern's data, it was highly skewed toward sensitivity. Almost every tumor demonstrated sensitivity in the laboratory, except a few. There was a small subset of patients whose tumors grew under any and all circumstances. These were the patients with the highest degree (extreme) drug resistance (EDR).

I immediately went about testing this hypothesis by reexamining our lung cancer data. Using this approach, I showed and reported that a small subset of lung cancer patients appeared to have a high degree of resistance to all the commonly used drugs. This was reported at the American Association for Cancer Research meetings and served as the basis for a research grant that I submitted in 1990 (Nagourney 1990).

Oddly, the concept of EDR seemed more appealing to the medical community. They had already taken to heart the idea that chemosensitivity assays weren't good at finding drugs, but believed that they were reasonably good at eliminating them. For them, EDR was a comfortable departure from their usual arguments about the ineffectiveness of chemosensitivity testing. This wasn't chemosensitivity after all, it was chemoresistance.

I was amused by the fact that this revisioning won over the critics. For the time being, I promoted Oncotech's EDR assay and we published a series of papers. But, deep down, I knew that it was wrong. I knew that growing cancer cells and measuring what stopped them from growing was ultimately of little importance. I knew that this tortured logic was little more than a dying paradigm clinging to life. And I knew that I wanted to get out of Oncotech.

I didn't like the business management, I didn't trust the science, and I couldn't, for the life of me, figure out how to use a laboratory test whose sole purpose was to tell you what not to do.

You don't go to the airport to find out where the airline isn't flying. You don't go to a restaurant to find out what they aren't serving. And cancer patients don't go to their doctors to find out what *not* to take. I needed clinically relevant answers for my patients. They needed to know what was going to work for them. And I wanted to know how to develop and apply new therapies.

Oncotech and its laboratory platform, based on cell growth, couldn't do it.

It is said that there are several happiest days in your life. The day you're married, the day that your children are born and, for me, the day I left Oncotech.

4

Anything That Works

Among the readership of this book perhaps there are physicians who no doubt remember the prodigious amount of work that we as first- and second-year medical students were forced to endure. Despite that workload, I can recall the pleasure of taking an occasional Saturday afternoon off.

As a send-off for medical school, my father had kindly provided me with subscriptions to the *New Yorker* and *The Saturday Review*. A couple of weekends each month, I indulged myself with the guilty pleasure of relaxing on my bed and reading nonmedical literature. One afternoon, as the sun was beginning to set, I came upon an article in *The Saturday Review* by Norman Cousins. An accomplished journalist and recognized author, Cousins, the magazine's editor, had penned an article titled "Anatomy of an Illness: As Perceived by the Patient" (later a book by the same title). He described his battle with anklyosing spondylitis, a debilitating autoimmune disease that results in a loss of flexibility so extreme that patients are soon wheelchair-bound. There are no cures for anklyosing spondylitis and in the 1970s there were few treatments. With such a dismal prognosis, Cousins devised a treatment regime consisting of vitamin C and a large helping of laughter provided by the regular viewing of Marx Brothers movies.

His response to these relatively simple interventions was nothing short of remarkable—allowing him to return to normal activities, free of the signs and symptoms associated with this devastating disease. I remember, as I read the article, wondering to myself whether these simple ministrations could provide the real, objective clinical benefit that Cousins described. How remarkable it would be, I thought, to avoid the toxicities, hazards, and expense of synthetic drugs, replacing them with these simple lifestyle changes. That article had an important impact on my thinking. It challenged my heretofore unwavering belief in allopathic medicine and forced me to confront the possible legitimacy of what came to be known years later as complementary alternative medicine (CAM). This would be a topic to which I would return many times in the course of my career.

Physicians have long referred to their craft as "the healing arts." I find the term appealing for it encompasses well-being in the context of a multitude of skill sets. Physicians often forget that we are the descendants of the shamans. With few medicines at their disposal, the shamans relied upon their healing powers. Chinese and Ayurvedic medicines both applied medicaments extracted from natural products. While there are many therapeutic substances found in these remedies, they are often combined with acupuncture, acupressure, aromatherapy, massage, yoga, laying on of hands, Qigong, music, and meditation. In the truest sense, the *healing arts* combine all these processes to provide the best possible outcome for each patient. Why has modern medicine eschewed these supportive measures?

As discovery favors a prepared mind, my encounter with Dr. Alan Kapuler, the gifted scientist who is the subject of chapter 12, enabled me to reexamine the many aspects of complementary care that he applied so successfully in the management of his own disease. While it is beyond the scope of this book to describe all of the disciplines that fall under the rubric of CAM, it is instructive to highlight some of the areas that I have incorporated into my practice.

Among the themes that course through the body of this book,

one concept arises repeatedly: metabolism, that collection of chemical and physical processes that sustain life and metabolomics, the study thereof. It has long been my belief that cancer is a metabolic disease and that the genetics of cancer are little more than the repository of information that metabolically active organisms draw upon to create the enzymes necessary for the production of energy. "You are what you eat," a catchphrase from the sixties, may turn out to be more prescient than we realized. The dictates of an indirect proof stipulate that if A = B and B = C, then A = C. Extending this reasoning in the biosphere: if food equals energy and energy equals life, then food equals life. And, by inference, if cancer is a metabolic disorder and metabolic disorders are changes in energy production, then cancer is a disease of changed energy production. For better or worse, our success as living organisms reflects the degree to which we shepherd and support cellular bioenergetic functions, most of which take place within the organelle known as the mitochondrian. Be good to your mitochondria and they will be good to you.

As the power of modern technology is finally applied to the root cause of most illnesses, we will discover that diet and lifestyle are the fundamentals of health.

There is a growing recognition that all diseases have a metabolic basis. We know, for example, that heart health equals cancer prevention. Appropriate management of blood lipids and maintenance of blood sugar, consumption of soy products, and regular exercise have been shown to reduce not only cardiovascular risk, but cancer risks in the form of prostate, breast, uterine, and other malignancies. Investigators like Mark Moyad, MD, from the Department of Urology at the University of Michigan, are now engaged in the study of statins and, more recently, metformin (the blood sugar–lowering agent) for their capacities to reduce prostate cancer incidence.

During my study of garlic as a medicinal, described in chapter 13, a basic concept of human dietary habits slowly came into focus. As I pondered man's consumption of garlic, and its broad appeal across diverse societies, I realized that we do not eat specific foods and spices because they taste good; instead, they taste good because they're good for us. Humankind has evolved around the food supply. Our developed frontal cortex and keen vision enabled us to identify needed foodstuffs in the canopy of the forest and to remember their location and seasonality from year to year. Similarly, we came to enjoy garlic, turmeric, rosemary, and other spices for their salubrious properties.

Even the most mundane of foodstuffs reflect healthful sources of micronutrients. That yellow mustard on your hot dog is an excellent source of selenium, magnesium, manganese, thiamin, and omega-3 fatty acids. Pickle relish contains carotenoids and lutein, as well as dietary fiber. The pickling process itself provides lactate and vinegar. Ketchup is a good source of lycopene and carotenoids. Indeed, the widely recognized metric for antioxidant activity, the Trolox equivalent antioxidant capacity (TEAC), recognizes ketchup as a potent free radical scavenger.

There are few Americans today who are not current or former members of a gym. The fitness craze is well established in the United States. Yet, few people realize the biochemical impact of physical activity upon health. Exercise induces changes in cellular physiology that have far-reaching effects. Above and beyond the obvious cardiac fitness, effects upon bone density, and well-being associated with endorphin release, are its very profound influence upon cellular metabolism. Muscular activity demands a ready source of energy. To meet this need the cell alters glucose uptake and metabolism, mitochondrial function, and insulin signaling. At the center of this process is a key enzyme known as AMP kinase. Sitting at the crossroads of all metabolic activity, this enzyme regulates the quantities of ATP (the primary source of energy for all life) drawing upon all intracellular sources of energy. It is alterations in this enzyme and its close partner LKB-1 that underlie the metabolic syndrome, diabetes, cardiovascular disease, and cancer. Through the action of AMP kinase and its downstream signaling, exercise doesn't just make us feel better, it makes us better.

As a third-year medical student, one of my classmates was conducting basic research on the neurotransmitter catecholamines for their impact upon lymphocyte signaling. He asked if I would volunteer by providing him 10cc of blood and offered to pay me $10 for my participation. While, as I recall, he never actually paid me the $10, I remember our conversation as he drew my blood.

"Catecholamine signaling in lymphocytes?" I said, as the blood drained into the green-topped tube.

"Yes," he said, as he looked up. "After all, the brain is a lymphocyte."

I remember the encounter well. Here I was sitting at the Royal Victoria Hospital in Montreal, just blocks from one of the fathers of psychoneuroimmunology, Hans Selye, MD. Dr. Selye, while at the University of Montreal, was among the first to conceive of emotional stress causing disability. His work on the general adaptation syndrome described adrenal hypertrophy, gastric ulceration, and immune deficiency as the byproducts of chronic stress. Subsequent work has defined the close association between the sympathetic nervous system (catecholamines), the hypothalamic-pituitary-adrenal axis, and the disruption of homeostasis that can predispose humans to such varied illnesses as cardiovascular disease, Parkinson's disease, the metabolic syndrome, and cancer.

Increasingly sophisticated experiments have now established a link between stress and the function of lymphocytes, as well as their responsiveness to antigens. With our growing recognition that cancer arises under conditions of physical and possibly emotional stress, psychological and social adaptations remain an important focus for future research.

The dizzying array of treatment options now available to cancer patients can leave these unsuspecting individuals prey for unscrupulous practitioners. What diet? What nutrient? What lifestyle change?

Into the fray, a small number of dedicated investigators have begun to provide these answers.

One such individual is Ralph Moss, PhD, former science writer for Memorial Sloan-Kettering Cancer Center. In his *Moss Reports* he provides rigorous analyses of the data that supports or, in some circumstances, does not support, alternative cancer treatments. As an arbiter of scientific legitimacy, Dr. Moss travels the world visiting and interviewing purveyors of treatment programs that fall outside the purview of conventional Western practices. He endeavors to understand the methods and materials of each practitioner and provides an honest assessment of their merits. He scrupulously avoids any possible conflict between himself and those he reviews, providing unbiased material to patients in need.

Among the physicians who have made a study of integrative oncologic care is Keith Block, MD, medical director, Block Center for Integrated Cancer Treatment and director of Integrated Medical Education, University of Illinois College of Medicine. Dr. Block has championed the concept of integrative cancer treatments. He defines a person's successful response to illness as the intersection of improved lifestyle, boosting biologic competence, and enhancing treatment options. He views cancer management as a continuum that begins with an attack phase, followed by a containment phase, and finally a maintenance phase. Combining diet, exercise, and the reduction of oxidative stress and inflammation he has developed an attractive program for cancer patients.

During my oncology fellowship at Georgetown University I had a discussion with an accomplished Serbian physician who was on a research sabbatical at the Lombardi Cancer Center. He was part of a tradition of scientific clinicians and he had come to the United States to expand his skills and technical capabilities. I always enjoyed my discussions with him for he brought a perspective that I did not often encounter with my American colleagues, an almost childlike inquisitiveness and sense of joy at discovery. He told me one evening that he thought I had the capacity to make discoveries. I was flattered and asked, "Why?" He said, because a discoverer must be eclectic. Eclecticism, the capacity to draw upon disparate disciplines, has been a guiding principle for me ever since. I describe my medical activities in one slightly humorous catchphrase. When asked by my patients and colleagues what it is I do, I respond, "I give conventional treatments unconventionally and give unconventional treatments conventionally." This principle has continued to be a guiding light for me as a physician.

5

The Neutrino

Every second, 300 billion solar neutrinos pass through every square inch of every human body on earth. And, for most of recorded history, we knew absolutely nothing about them.

In 1930, particle physicist Wolfgang Pauli, while working on the nuclear reaction known as beta decay, suggested that a small subatomic particle of specific dimension and velocity must exist. Several years later, Enrico Fermi coined the term "neutrino," or "little neutral one," to describe this uncharged particle.

Although the technology did not exist to measure or identify the particles, both Pauli and Fermi absolutely, positively knew they existed. They based their conclusion on one of the most fundamental principle in physics—the conservation of momentum. They knew that if a positive particle and a negative particle traveled away from the nuclear reaction there had to be another particle that they could not see that traveled in a different direction to balance the mass and velocity forces (momentum).

In 1956, Clyde L. Cowan Jr., PhD, and colleagues used the method for the measurement of subatomic particles, beta capture, to detect neutrinos, an accomplishment that decades later led to the Nobel Prize. Neither Pauli nor Fermi ever wavered from their position; it just took sixty-five years for the scientific community to recognize what they had done.

ANOTHER SCIENTIFIC MYSTERY

When I first became interested in chemosensitivity testing in the early 1980s, I had never taken the time to consider what it was I was actually measuring. It seemed obvious. Cancers overtook their hosts, drugs were designed to stop the process, and adding drugs into a tissue culture tube enabled me to pick the winners.

Working with Dr. Weisenthal, I had adopted his laboratory test that measured whether cells lived or died following a drug exposure. This was a departure from the measurement of cell growth and its inhibition—the predominant technology of that time.

My choice of cell death measures was originally predicated on the greater speed and efficiency that they offered over the rather cumbersome, slow, and inefficient clonogenic technique. As my experience grew, however, I became convinced that there was something very different about measuring cancer cell death compared with measuring cancer cell growth. Like a melody lingering in my mind, or an itch I couldn't scratch, I pondered the cell-death/cell-growth dichotomy every day as I worked in my lab.

With each clinical success, I became more convinced of the merit of cell death measures. Despite the protestations of my scientific and clinical colleagues, who had abandoned the field in droves following the 1983 *NEJM* article, I knew with every fiber of my being that what I did worked. I just didn't know why.

During those dark days of the mid-1980s, no one believed that you could use human cancer cells to select drugs. After all, the *NEJM* had said so. The medical and scientific communities had seen that it didn't work and, by extension, reasoned that it could never work. My good outcomes were viewed as chance events while my presentations at professional meetings were met with polite disinterest.

During that period of time, I used my technique in collaboration with a laboratory technologist named Rick Kyle. He was using the clonogenic assay to study drug combinations and synergy. While he was a career scientist, I was a medical fellow spending a year in the laboratory. As such, he viewed my results with a modicum of disdain. Yet, it was I who made the observation that 5-FU was synergistic with alpha-interferon, an observation that we subsequently published together. Years later, the interaction between interferon and an enzyme named thymidine phosphorylase explained what we had found so many years before.

Like the discovery of the neutrino, before it could be captured and quantified, I knew that cell death studies held insights that would someday help to explain many of cancer's mysteries. I just couldn't put my finger on why.

The French philosopher Rene Descartes said, *"Cogito ergo sum."* Translated, it means, "I think, therefore I am." Descartes believed that his senses were true, his observations real, and that this was proof of his existence.

I repeated my experiments over and over. I checked for errors. I examined for possible artifacts. I documented every experiment, working evenings and weekends, manually calculating every study. I could not find an error in my reasoning. My patients' remissions were my neutrinos. There was an explanation for my successes. I just didn't have a "beta capture experiment" to prove it yet.

That would occur in 1992 when I would hear Alan Eastman, PhD, from Dartmouth College describe the phenomenon and implications of apoptosis (a form of programmed cell death). Suddenly, it would all make perfect sense.

6

Epiphany

I was returning home from the 1992 American Association for Cancer Research meeting in San Diego and decided to leave early to avoid traffic. By the time I hit Del Mar it was fairly clear sailing on the northbound 5 freeway.

My poster presentation the prior day coincided with a special symposium that I had desperately wished to attend. Cochaired by Dr. Alan Eastman, it was a discussion of hormone and chemotherapy response in cells. Unable to attend, I purchased the audiotape of the session and popped it into my rented Thunderbird's cassette player as I headed north.

Despite the relatively poor quality of the tape, with paper shuffling and echoes in the background, the information struck me like a bolt of lightning. It started with a discussion by a German investigator on cyproterone acetate, a synthetic hormone used for the treatment of advanced prostate cancer. Like other hormonal therapies, cyproterone acetate could induce dramatic responses in patients. Dr. Eastman then began the discussion of the chemotherapy drug cisplatin. Developed in the 1970s, this drug was believed to inhibit DNA use in the process of mitosis (cell division). With each passing lecture, the theme became clearer. Whatever the drugs were designed to do—hormone withdrawal, DNA damage, or inhibition of cell division—they worked by forcing cells to undergo a process of programmed cell death.

Each lecturer returned repeatedly to the term "apoptosis." Apoptosis, from the Greek, was coined by investigators in England who recognized that every cell in a multicellular organism carries with it an "off" switch. Like leaves falling from a deciduous tree at the end of the growing season, cells no longer capable of providing the function for which they were designed are eliminated neatly, cleanly, and permanently. Apoptosis, or "controlled cell deletion," served as the body's executioner for errant cells.

It seems that multicellular existence reflects a cellular social contract. Every cell is granted protection, mobility, oxygen, and nutritional support. In return every cell must serve the body as a whole. When a cell is damaged, injured, irradiated, or infected by a virus, the grim reaper slices it to bits and presents it to the immune system for dinner. Doing the dirty work are nuclear enzymes known as caspases. These essential proteins found in every human cell have been preserved since the origin of the most primordial multicellular organisms. Indeed, the proteins engaged in human cell death are virtually the same as the enzymes found in the roundworm (*Caenrhabdtis elegans*). It was the work of H. Robert Horvitz, MD, on this species that lead to the 2002 Nobel Prize in medicine, confirming the relevance of programmed cell death in human physiology and cancer therapeutics.

All at once, I got it. Like a bolt of lightning, I was struck. The answers to questions that I had been asking for ten years were right there in front of me. Suddenly, it all made sense.

This is why killing cells accurately predicted patients' outcomes, while all the other assays didn't work. Of course they didn't work. They couldn't work—you could never, ever predict a patient's response to a drug based on that drug's ability to stop cells from growing. It was utterly and completely irrelevant. No wonder the clonogenic and all the other assays measuring growth didn't work— they couldn't. I GOT IT!

I stopped the tape, rewound, and listened over and over again. Dr. Eastman described his work and while I couldn't gauge the accuracy of his suggested mechanism, I knew beyond a shadow of a doubt that a cell's response to effective drugs was quick and deadly. Cancer cells didn't grow too much, they died too little. Apoptosis and programmed cell death explained it all.

SHARING MY REVELATION

I arrived at my apartment in Long Beach to find my older brother, Brian, visiting from Santa Barbara. I burst in the door, rabid with my new insight.

I was like the telephone lineman played by Richard Dreyfuss in the film *Close Encounters of the Third Kind,* re-creating a mountain in his living room from mental images seared into his brain by an alien force. I was possessed. I rambled on in a fugue state to my unsuspecting brother. I couldn't talk fast enough. Ten years of wandering in the desert. Ten years of senior investigators denigrating my work. Ten years of manuscripts turned down repeatedly. Ten years of failed grant applications. Suddenly, it all made sense.

We were measuring something completely different. We hadn't found a new route to India; we had unsuspectingly discovered the new world. The world of programmed cell death, apoptosis, and DNA degradation. This was the world in which damaged, mutated, and abnormal cells killed themselves in service to the organism as a whole. Chemotherapy didn't murder cells—it convinced them to commit suicide.

No wonder bone marrow transplants didn't work. No wonder complex, dose-intense drug combinations couldn't cure patients. It was obvious; the cancer cells didn't speak their language. If the cells spoke Adriamycin (a commonly used chemotherapy), comparatively low doses would prove effective. However, if the cell doesn't speak Cytoxan (another widely used chemotherapy), then no amount could cure the patient.

When American tourists find themselves frustrated by their Parisian waiters, their first response is always to shout. But, if someone, or for that matter a cell, doesn't speak your language, no amount of shouting (dose intensity) can help. The failure of certain drugs to eliminate cancer cells in vitro (in a test tube, e.g.) and the ability of other drugs to obliterate cells at the lowest possible concentrations all made sense. I could achieve with a whisper what others could not do with a bullhorn, so long as I chose my language carefully in the laboratory.

I went over and over it again with my poor brother. No one believed in it before, but now I knew why it worked. I felt certain that I would explain this to the naysayers and they would immediately accept all of that accumulated data. I was convinced they would listen now.

7

Cell Death Allows for Life

Programmed cell death and its implications for cancer biology are at the core of this book. But programmed cell death was not "invented" in 1948 when nitrogen mustard (the first chemotherapy) was discovered, nor was it first explored in the 1990s when I first learned of it.

Long before cancer, long before human beings, the process of programmed cell death existed to regulate cell behavior in multicellular organisms. We can trace, through genetic analysis, the evolution of human caspase proteins all the way back to the roundworm. In each instance these grim reapers are designed to cull the herd of the sick and weak. The process that winnows out the damaged cell leaves the organism as a whole all the stronger. It is not the cancer cell that outgrows its counterparts, which strikes fear into the heart of every organism, but instead the cancer cell that outlives its normal counterparts and survives to divide another day. Fearing the implications of such mutinous behavior, complex organisms have developed assassins to silently smite their long-lived enemies.

If it isn't cancer that apoptosis was put in place for, what is it? The easiest examples of physiological apoptosis can be found during embryogenesis and development in utero. The human hand, for example, with five digits, begins life as a mitt, a thumb and four fused fingers. As we mature, during the process of gestation, the body, under a carefully constructed genetic code, dissolves away the tissue

43

between the digits allowing the dexterity needed to function as a human. Perhaps you have encountered someone in your own life with a webbed toe—a "nonmalignant" example of the failure of apoptosis.

More striking is the example of sexual dimorphism. Human beings, under the control of their X and Y chromosomes, diverge several weeks into gestation into male or female. Before this gender commitment occurs, however, both male and female genitalia arise, the former as the Wolffian duct and the latter as the Mullerian duct. If the child carries a Y chromosome (the determinate of maleness in the human) then the body produces a substance known as Mullerian inhibitory factor (MIF), which actively "kills off" the Mullerian traits (uterus, ovary, cervix) allowing the Wolffian attributes to mature (penis, testicles, prostate).

Thus, you don't just become a male; you must first actively kill off the female within you. The same process occurs in reverse if an XX chromosomal makeup is found. The failure of this gender determination results in births with ambiguous genitalia. As there is no true hermaphroditism in humans (that is, both reproductively male and female), the physical attributes associated with these common birth defects are little more than the failure to kill off the physical features, not the biological. Indeed, ambiguous genitalia is not an uncommon birth defect and is usually corrected shortly after birth.

APOPTOSIS FOR LIFE

Above and beyond developmental biology, why would we, into adulthood, continue to rely on active apoptotic responses? The answer to this leads us to cancer and carcinogenesis. While it was not appreciated some decades ago, we now realize that infectious diseases are an important cause of cancer.

Among the causative factors are common viral infections. Viruses, for all their simplicity (a protein coat, small amount of genetic material, and an apparatus that enables them to inject their information into a cell), are pretty intelligent. They know that the human body is on guard protecting itself against invasion. Swarming through the bloodstream are lymphocytes, prepared at a moment's notice to paint the viruses with proteins known as antibodies and laser-guide the immune shock troops, macrophages and polymorphonuclear leukocytes (polys), to engulf them. Should a virus escape detection and successfully invade a cell, apoptosis comes to the rescue.

Viruses are not, in the truest sense of the word, "alive." They have no metabolic activity. To exist at all, they must invade a living cell. Using only their genetic information, which they pump through the membrane of the cell, allowing it to reach the nucleus, they take over the cell's machinery and use it to produce new viruses; not just one or two, but hundreds, even thousands. Confronted by these marauding hijackers, with the enemy already within the walls and the safety of the entire organism in peril, the cell does the only thing left to it—it kills itself and shuts down the very process that allows the virus to propagate and succeed.

The signals that tell the cell it's under assault from its very deepest reaches are a collection of proteins that function like a genomic checkout clerk. For anyone who has ever inadvertently (or otherwise) attempted to walk out of a store with a package that contains a magnetic strip, you'll know the alarms go off, and the store guard descends. You're not allowed through the checkout line and out of the store unless the clerk approves your passage.

Similarly, cells are not allowed to go through cell division unless their genes are "clean." By "clean" I mean free of mutation and viral inclusions. The virus, after all, must insinuate itself into your genetic makeup in order to commandeer the machinery. By wedging itself into your chromosomes, the virus flags the checkout clerk and declares its presence. It is only by disarming the magnetic-strip reader that the virus is allowed to play. Thus, disarming the most profound protective mechanisms of each cell is essential for viral success.

Over the eons that this cat-and-mouse game has been played, viruses have become increasingly clever. With each defense marshaled by a cell, the virus learns to cloak itself in ever more nefarious costumes. When the cell activates the p53 genomic integrity gene (a tumor suppressor gene), the virus anticipates the move by synthesizing a protein known as E6, which binds and deactivates the defense. When the cell then sends a retinoblastoma (RB) protein into the mix, the virus responds with an E7 protein and shuts down this checkout clerk's magnetic device. One by one, the cell's defenses are laid to waste and the viruses are allowed to duplicate. All the viruses want to do, in a manner of speaking, is raise a family and protect themselves from the cell's desire to commit suicide. The inadvertent result of the virus's success, however, is the disarming of the cell's ability to detect and respond to mutation. Unwittingly, the virus has opened up the floodgate to malignant transformation, all driven by a loss of apoptotic response.

Many people have heard of the human papilloma virus (HPV) of which there are many subtypes. The viral infection that results in venereal warts disarms the body, allowing, as an unintended consequence, the cancerous transformation that ultimately kills the host. Here, in an infectious context, is the process fundamental to malignant transformation. Any mutation that eliminates a cell's ability to die sets in motion the development of cancer.

For the virus, cancer is an unintended consequence of the virus's capacity to self-servingly undermine the cell's apoptotic capacity. Not surprisingly, many mutations that lead to cancer arise in these same cell-death pathways.

Benzopyrene, a common constituent of cigarette smoke, damages the p53 gene resulting in cigarette-smoke–associated lung cancer. The childhood brain tumors associated with retinoblastoma result from mutations in this critical cell-death regulatory protein. Indeed, the complete loss of p53 function in a rare disorder known as Li-Fraumeni syndrome results in death by cancer usually by the second decade, with the average victim suffering between three to five separate and distinct malignancies. Thus, alterations in survival signals are the paramount change in cancer and the reason why the dictum "cancer doesn't grow too much, it dies too little" rings true.

8

Unraveling the Mystery

In 1992, I was the director of experimental therapeutics at Long Beach Memorial Medical Center. I had a great lab, great staff, and a wealth of interesting data. With chronic lymphocytic leukemia, my principal model for experimentation, I was slowly unraveling the mystery of programmed cell death. When did it happen? Why did it happen? How did it happen? What caused it? Was it only chemotherapy and radiation, or would biological materials like the immune system toxin, tumor necrosis factor, have the same effect?

In collaboration with Dr. Weisenthal, we had previously completed our "first proof of concept" study. Beginning in 1983, in collaboration with the Pediatric Oncology Group at Long Beach Memorial Medical Center, blood samples and bone marrow aspirates from children newly diagnosed with acute lymphoblastic leukemia (ALL) were submitted for drug response evaluation. This cancer, the leading cause of cancer death in children, had been managed successfully with corticosteroids for decades. Cortisone, prednisone, and dexamethasone were the mainstays of therapy and provided prompt, but generally brief, remissions.

I remember vividly, when I was a small child, that my older cousin Liam was treated for this disease. His face blew up like a balloon, the characteristic side effect of these therapies (known as "chipmunk facies"). Despite his brief remission, he too died from this disease and I attended his funeral. Here we were, twenty years later, and children were still dying at the same rate.

Dr. Weisenthal and I reasoned that the outcome of children with ALL was less dependent on *what* they received and more a function of *who* received it. That is, some children had the capacity to respond to therapy and others did not. It followed that sensitivity to the corticosteroids (known to induce apoptosis as their mode of action) in the laboratory could divide children into the good- and bad-responding groups and, possibly, predict their survival.

Every new sample of leukemia was tested against dexamethasone at one micro molar (the concentration of exposure in the test tube). Their leukemic blasts (the most immature form, the stem cell of a leukemia process) either died or they didn't. Patients were categorized as dexamethasone-sensitive and dexamethasone-resistant. We were kept unaware (blinded) of the children's outcome and the treating physicians were kept unaware (blinded) to our results. We reasoned that the children found sensitive in vitro would have the best survivals, while those found resistant would have the worst. And then we broke the code and examined the accuracy of our predictions.

The results were astonishing. The children whose blast cells all died in the test tube following four days of dexamethasone exposure all remained in remission without relapse at their five-year follow-up; those children whose blast cells appeared resistant continued to relapse, with only 25 percent of those children still alive at five years. A middle group fell in between. In essence, we knew four days after diagnosis which children would live and which children would die.

We submitted the paper to the *NEJM* and several years later went on to report our initial observations at the apoptosis meetings in San Diego and the International Drug Resistance Symposium in Amsterdam. Despite the warm reception that we received from the scientists in La Jolla and those in Holland, the editors of the *NEJM* turned down the paper. As did the editors of *Leukemia* and every other journal to which I submitted the manuscript. Somehow, my enthusiasm for apoptosis wasn't proving very contagious.

While the basic scientists rapidly grasped the implications of these observations, the clinicians turned a blind eye. I was disappointed by the reception from our clinical colleagues, but I knew that we were on to something very important.

During the next several years, we drilled down into the phenomenon of apoptosis, examining the biochemistry and molecular biology using sophisticated tools like flow cytometry and DNA gel electrophoresis. The field was becoming increasingly complicated, with new parameters described almost every day. I began to wonder what would be the best measure of programmed cell death. And then a colleague and collaborator from Australia published a paper in *Cancer Research* in 1994. He compared a variety of measures and concluded that the most accurate, reliable, reproducible, and dependable gauge of programmed cell death was "delayed loss of membrane integrity." This was the process, over several days, by which the barrier between the inside of the cell and outside (membrane) disintegrated resulting in the loss of cellular viability.

My God, I thought. This was precisely where I had begun my work in the first place—using stains to measure the loss of membrane integrity in a process we call the differential staining technique. Dr. Weisenthal and I had been right all along and hadn't realized it.

While many measures might work in pure cell systems like cell lines, and even some cancers like leukemia, this same staining technique would prove immensely valuable as my work moved from the blood-borne tumors to the much more common and deadly solid tumors like colon, lung, and pancreas.

I remained at Long Beach Memorial Medical Center until the hospital eliminated its basic cancer research program. On July 1, 1995, Steve Evans, MA, chief technical officer; Young Zhuang Su, MD, senior scientist; and I pulled up stakes and moved our operations to a small, midcentury structure on the corner of Elm Avenue and 36th Street in Long Beach.

After months of structural revision, equipment purchases, and quality assessments, regulatory approval was finally achieved and our laboratory was fully operational. Rational Therapeutics, however difficult its gestation, was born.

9

Finally, Rational Therapy

O ne evening in 1995, while I was working on the oncology unit at Long Beach Memorial, I received an unexpected phone call at about 6:30 PM from New York. I say "unexpected" because I didn't normally receive calls from patients on the oncology ward after hours. For some reason, I did so on this particular night, and I could never have foreseen that the man on the other end of the line would make an extraordinary impact on me and my practice.

The caller introduced himself as Wayne Atwood. He was a patient on the leukemia service of Memorial Sloan-Kettering (MSK) Cancer Center in New York City and was undergoing therapy for acute promyelocytic leukemia (APL).

I well understood a diagnosis of APL. This type of leukemia carries a chromosomal translocation (a break in the DNA that moves a piece of one chromosome and attaches it to a different chromosome some distance away) known as the t(15;17). Patients with this type tend to respond to a class of drugs known as retinoids (derivatives of vitamin A). Wayne had initially shown good response to this class of drugs but did not benefit from the subsequent chemotherapy administered in the form of consolidation (intense therapy designed to enhance the benefit of treatment).

Wayne had seen national network television coverage of my work that included a dramatic story of a young man with a very resist-

51

ant leukemia who had sent a blood sample to our laboratory from Nevada. That patient achieved an unexpectedly good remission from an unusual three-drug combination, and Wayne was hoping for a similarly good outcome.

Wayne explained that he had just completed a standard two-drug combination known as 3 plus 7. Regrettably, his bone marrow still showed persistent leukemia. He wasn't responding, yet his doctor was planning to give him exactly the same thing all over again.

I pondered Wayne's situation and felt convinced that something else needed to be done. When I asked him what the rationale for repeating the exact same drugs might be, he explained that the young physician was "just following orders." As I sat at the unit's nursing station considering Wayne's dilemma, I recall specifically what I told him over the phone in response: "Your physician doesn't have a stake in your outcome."

After all, I reasoned, whether or not Wayne got better, there would always be another patient to treat with APL. But for Wayne, he couldn't afford to continue on this medical merry-go-round. Each cycle of therapy carried known toxicities, risks of infection and bleeding, and cost him precious time.

I said, "Wayne, why don't you make a deal with your doctor? Tell him that you will accept his recommendation. If it works, he will be proven correct and capable as a physician and his judgment will be vindicated. However, if it does not work, you will receive in return his firstborn."

My colleague, Jonathan Blitzer, MD, overheard our conversation. I don't recall his exact comments, but he was somewhere between bemused and shocked by my candid vilification of this physician's random application of chemotherapies. I told Wayne that I would do things differently. He paused for a moment and replied, "In that case, Dr. Nagourney, I'll see you tomorrow."

Wayne Atwood and his wife, Linette, were successful convention newspaper and magazine publishers from Kansas City. They arrived in California the next day, making them the first official visitors to my new clinic. Wayne was young, energetic, and bright, with his charming and lovely wife, Linette, by his side. Their nearly five-year-old daughter Carly was back at the hotel. Wayne couldn't wait to get started with treatment.

I conducted a bone marrow aspiration (the process by which a needle is inserted into the pelvic bone and the marrow contained within is suctioned out through a syringe) and used a centrifuge to isolate the leukemic blasts, which were plentiful in his case. We studied a large number of drugs and combinations; to my surprise and delight I found that Wayne remained very sensitive to the original drug known as ATRA (All Trans Retinoic Acid). Better still, he was sensitive to several other comparatively mild drugs.

Our mission became clear and focused: We had to find the chemotherapy combination that would clear his bone marrow of the leukemic blasts and get him back in remission. In doing so Wayne would qualify for a brand-new experimental protocol back at MSK. The study used a new monoclonal antibody (an immune protein) directed against a cell surface protein called CD33. This was a "smart bomb" against the leukemic stem cell and had the possibility of helping him, but we first needed a complete remission.

We placed an IV access port in his chest, started him on an oral vitamin A derivative (ATRA), and infused the mild chemotherapeutics identified in the laboratory assay. Wayne felt so well on therapy that he checked out of the hospital and received most of the rest of his treatments poolside at the Long Beach Marriott hotel. A week went by, Carly played in the pool, Linette managed their thriving publishing business from across the country, and Wayne's leukemia cells disappeared—almost without toxicity. The second bone marrow was normal. Wayne was in remission. Success!

The microscope slides were prepared and readied for transfer to New York. I contacted the senior investigator at MSK and requested that they accrue Wayne to the trial.

Upon Wayne's return to New York, his physicians were pleased with the remission. The senior physician nodded approvingly, suggesting to Wayne that there was just the slightest glimmer of acceptance of our approach. But the junior physician, from behind closed doors said to Wayne, "I'll accrue you to the anti-CD33 protocol, but lose the charlatan in California." I can still see Wayne's laughing eyes and knowing smile as he confided that professional "secret" to me during our next visit.

Wayne did very well for several years. We lost the typical doctor-patient relationship, became good friends, and corresponded regularly. He and Linette would visit when they were in California. After several years, however, a relapse occurred. Wayne contacted us and sent a bone marrow sample from Texas, where he was undergoing evaluation under the care of Karel Dicke, MD, PhD, an accomplished stem cell transplantation expert.

Dr. Dicke was willing to allow us to assist in the selection of the bone marrow preparation regimen. We conducted our analyses, paying close attention to the effect of higher and higher drug dosages (those associated with bone marrow transplant) and recommended a combination of alkylating agents and VP-16 (also known as etoposide).

Wayne achieved a remission and went on for another year or two. By this time, however, the recurrences were coming faster. It was increasingly difficult to identify active treatments. His stem cell reserves were compromised. His tolerance of therapy declined. Additional analyses identified fewer and fewer active drugs that his body would respond to favorably. His leukemia had become drug-resistant and, seven years after I met him, he succumbed to complications of his recurrent disease.

His two older sons were nearing adulthood and Carly was just eleven years old. Linette had come to realize this was one battle they couldn't win. I often wonder whether I might have been able to better control this disease had I met Wayne at the time of his diagnosis and prior to the onset of treatment.

Upon Wayne's passing, Linette felt a sense of commitment and obligation to other cancer patients and their families. She knew firsthand that the seven years Wayne survived didn't occur by chance. Wayne had made a determination that he would do everything possible to confront his cancer, that he would not take no for an answer. He would seek and find those doctors and investigators capable of providing solutions, leaving no stone unturned until he received the treatment that best matched his needs.

To facilitate patients' access to the most groundbreaking therapies, Linette went on to launch the *Patient Resource Cancer Guide*—a treatment and facilities guide published for patients and their families across the country. The catchphrase "Take Control" is emblazoned on the front cover of every issue. With a distinguished board of medical editors and advisors, this publication offers patients the opportunity to identify and pursue those options that offer the greatest chance of cure. In fact, Linette is so passionate about this cause that she makes the guides available free of charge upon request. You can order yours at www.PatientResource.net.

One year after her husband's death, Linette herself developed breast cancer and she requested our assistance. We identified the best treatments; she completed therapy and remains well and free of disease today. What perhaps best characterizes the Atwoods' approach to this difficult disease is a simple yet profound phrase found on the first page of each issue of the *Patient Resource Cancer Guide*—and a philosophy we at Rational Therapeutics truly believe in: "Effective self-advocacy begins with information." Indeed it does.

10

Never Give Cancer
an Even Break

When I am asked what it is we do for our cancer patients using laboratory-directed approaches, I say, "I cure the curable, treat the treatable, and avoid the toxicity and suffering of futile care." Our laboratory does not render incurable cancers curable, nor make untreatable patients treatable. It simply helps us figure out who is who before we treat them. One corollary to our principal approach is that curable cancers should be treated for cure the first time. Your best chance for remission or cure is always in the first-line setting. You never get a second chance at first-line chemotherapy.

One afternoon, I received a phone call from a young pulmonologist who had recently joined the staff at Long Beach Memorial Medical Center. The physician, Cameron Dick, MD, was smart, energetic, and aggressive, but we had never come to be especially close friends. On this particular afternoon he called me to discuss a case. A fifty-four-year-old gentleman had presented to his office with increasing shortness of breath. A chest x-ray revealed that the lower lobe of the left lung was collapsed. A subsequent biopsy showed small cell carcinoma of the lung.

Small cell lung cancer (SCLC; also known as oat cell carcinoma) is the most aggressive form of lung cancer. Usually arising in the center of the chest, it spreads rapidly. Without effective treatment it can be lethal within months. Its propensity for dissemination to liver, bones, brain, even bone marrow makes it among the most aggressive solid tumors that medical oncologists confront. Recognizing that this previously healthy gentleman had a small chance of survival, Dr. Dick said something to the patient, subsequently quoted to me, that I will always remember. He said, "If you were my father, there is only one person I would send you to to treat this cancer—Dr. Nagourney."

I remember this because I didn't think of myself as Dr. Dick's choice for oncologic referral. I found it surprisingly flattering and unexpected. It also proved fortuitous.

When David Hanbidge arrived at my office, he was more worried than symptomatic, but he was certainly symptomatic. I explained that my approach would be to conduct a formal biopsy of his tumor, if necessary, by surgery. That I would choose the most active combinations of drugs and that I would likely give them in sequence to achieve maximum reduction in his tumor burden. He was in trouble and he knew it; the problem was, so did I.

My colleague, Douglas McConnell, MD, removed the entire left lower lobe and provided adequate tissue for analysis. Good degrees of activity were noted for the most widely used chemotherapy combination: cisplatin plus VP-16. But, even better activity was noted for cisplatin plus topotecan, a combination that would not become mainstream for three more years. Additional activity for cisplatin plus gemcitabine offered yet another opportunity for this patient, should we be fortunate enough to achieve a good remission.

Knowing up front that the patient would respond well, I opted to apply an aggressive radiation program given twice a day (as opposed to the usual once per day) and combined it with cisplatin plus VP-16 chemotherapy. Before we began treatment, I told David that in the eyes of most beholders, he had an incurable cancer. I went on to tell him that I had every intention of curing it. The one caveat was that this was going to be the most unpleasant six months of his life. I offered him the chance to seek other opinions. He declined.

"Hold on to your hat, David, you're not going to like this. But if everything goes right, when it's all over, you're going to like it a great deal."

Twice-a-day chest radiation with chemotherapy is no picnic. Consolidation with topotecan-based chemotherapy combined with low-dose brain radiation is worse. The brain radiation known as PCI (prophylactic cranial irradiation) was often used to prevent the development of brain metastases, while the topotecan combination was not. But the coup de grace was after every last remnant of measurable disease had long since disappeared, I came at him with a final series of cisplatin plus gemcitabine doublets, based upon his laboratory analysis to complete the job. It was a long, hard fight.

As the last waves of nausea from cisplatin therapy dissipated and David's mohawk haircut slowly grew in, I realized that he was in complete remission, and not any measure, not even the most sensitive biochemical parameter, revealed any evidence of disease: chromogranin A was normal; neuron-specific analysis was normal; his CEA, LDH, brain MRI, and chest/abdomen/pelvis CT scans were all normal. Indeed, they have all remained normal for twelve years. David Hanbidge is one of those rare, few individuals who can say, "I have been cured of SCLC."

Although I no longer follow David clinically, his chances of recurrence being so low, I do keep in touch and hear from him from time to time. An avid sailor, he and his wife enjoy an active lifestyle in Southern California. When I reflect on David's experience, several things come to mind. First, that all of the small cell lung cancer patients under my care who have been cured of their diseases received similar consolidation approaches (that is, non-cross-resistant drug combinations administered in sequence). Second, that curability is in the eye of the beholder. And, finally, that the repeated assault on cancer with different drugs and modalities (chemotherapy and radiation) can cure drug-sensitive diseases.

Is it possible that we could cure more small-cell lung cancer patients if we used similarly aggressive and intelligently directed approaches? That is something I hope to find out.

11

Outliving Hospice

In March 2005, Rick Carroll was undergoing evaluation to see if he qualified for "Pegasus," a new program at the VA Greater Los Angeles Healthcare System for the study and treatment of hepatitis C. During Rick's initial workup, an ultrasound of the abdomen was performed and a 6.5 cm mass was found on his right adrenal gland. A follow-up PET scan and chest x-ray revealed two masses in his left lung along with two lymph nodes that "lit up" on the PET scan. With a diagnosis of Stage IV non-small cell lung cancer (NSCLC), Rick went to Cedars-Sinai Medical Center for a second opinion.

After Cedars confirmed the diagnosis, the VA recommended carboplatin plus gemcitabine, a very appropriate therapy for Stage IV NSCLC. Rick responded only briefly to this treatment regime and by October of that year, his disease had begun to progress. Rick was sick, running daily fevers of up to 104 degrees, with severe night sweats, was unable to eat, and had subsequent weight loss. His physicians at the VA placed him first in the palliative care program and then ultimately on hospice.

But Rick was not going to go down without a fight. His girlfriend sent out a plea to friends and colleagues looking for answers. One of my former patients sent her information about our approach to therapy. Unbeknown to me, she contacted Rational Therapeutics and my staff put her in touch with Robert Shuman, MD, a thoracic surgeon, so a tumor sample could be obtained. During Rick's appointment with Dr. Shuman, he asked him straight out, "Just level with me, is this a waste of time?" Dr. Shuman told him, "No, it's not. I've seen Dr. Nagourney perform miracles."

One afternoon that November, I was making rounds on the sixth floor of Long Beach Memorial Medical Center, when a slender blonde woman stepped out of a room and introduced herself. "Hi, I'm Rick's sister Leinie. I just want to say how glad I am to meet you and how pleased we are to be here. When I heard Rick was having the surgery, I flew up from Florida to be with him. I am so impressed with the work you do."

I had absolutely no idea who this woman was; I had no idea who Rick was. I was only standing outside of this room because, as the director of the Todd Cancer Institute, I made a practice of meeting all patients on the oncology unit and Rick was one.

The nurse explained to me that Rick had come from Los Angeles to undergo a wedge resection under the care of Dr. Shuman after contacting Rational Therapeutics. Although my staff had referred him to Dr. Shuman to arrange for the biopsy in order to obtain a tumor sample, I had been unaware of his admission. So I walked into the room and introduced myself. A tall, slender man was lying in bed, recovering from a biopsy. He shook my hand, thanked me for my work, and told me he was looking forward to our results.

Rick's efforts were rewarded when we identified the unexpected combination of irinotecan plus cisplatin as a salvage regimen. The term "salvage" is applied in medicine, not unlike the nautical term for retrieving a sunken ship. Patients who have failed first- or second-line therapy, for whom options are limited, are given treatments in this context to "salvage" them from certain demise.

Riding his K1200 RS BMW motorcycle from West Los Angeles to Long Beach (thirty-five miles each way) Rick received his treatments on a two-weeks-on, one-week-off schedule. The ride on the motorcycle would take just long enough to get home before the side effects would start and he could head for bed. He would be sick for a couple of days, but as a business consultant he was able to carry on a full work schedule from home. All the while, the VA had already placed him on home-based terminal care known as hospice. Thankfully, Rick had just received a trust account and was drawing $20,000 a month, allowing him to cover the costs associated with the hospital stays and surgeries, as well as the doctor visits, treatments, medications, and supportive care.

In retrospect, it was well worth it, for he achieved a complete remission (the adrenal lesion had shrunk to the size of a raisin and no longer lit up on PET scan) that lasted a year. By the following fall, however, severe abdominal pain raised concerns.

Rick, in fact, had a large metastatic recurrence located deep within the abdomen in an area known as the retroperitoneal space.

Following his initial good response to carboplatin plus gemcitabine administered at the VA, Rick had proved himself to be a member of that small subset of patients who would respond well to second-line therapy (in this instance the combination of cisplatin plus irinotecan selected in the laboratory). Despite this, no one would seriously consider taking such a patient with a second relapse of metastatic lung cancer through an additional open biopsy. No one, that is, but me. Rick fully understood the risks and was prepared to proceed with the surgery and the repeat analysis. I explained to him that he was an "experiment" in real time. A tumor abutting the pancreas was removed and the pathology report verified that his original lung cancer had spread.

The hypothesis that I had been formulating for years suggested that the systematic elimination of cancer recurrences would ultimately render the patient free of disease. This was the embodiment of the chemotherapeutic approach that I had formulated years earlier during Dr. Steven Rosenberg's lecture on repeated surgeries for sarcoma (as noted in the preface).

As I see it, there are two plausible explanations for recurrent cancer in most patients. The first, represented by the school of drug-resistance investigators, holds that cancers mutate and acquire resistance as they are exposed to drug treatments. This spawned an active area of research spanning two decades during which oncologists, largely unsuccessfully, attempted to reverse drug resistance with calcium channel blocking agents and other drugs. The second explanation for drug resistance is one that reflects the outgrowth of tumor cell subpopulations that, from the very beginning, were insensitive to the drugs administered. Thus, a Darwinian selection process allows the outgrowth of inherently resistant clones.

I reasoned that if the latter were true, then the serial elimination of each subclone could ultimately lead to the absolute eradication of the cancer. If correct, Rick's November 2005 biopsy, which revealed resistance to cisplatin and gemcitabine (the treatment he had just failed), but showed sensitivity to irinotecan plus cisplatin, reflected clone #1 eliminated and clone #2 in the crosshairs.

With the cisplatin/irinotecan regimen now exhausted, would we find clone #3, with an entirely new profile of sensitivity? Indeed, that is exactly what we found. The tumor removed from the adrenal gland was now resistant to cisplatin plus gemcitabine, as well as cisplatin plus irinotecan. This new crop of cancer cells had unexpectedly come full circle to a profile of sensitivity for gefitinib (IRESSA), the new tyrosine kinase inhibitor, approved two years earlier for patients with NSCLC. With our studies in hand, we started Rick on the very closely related oral erlotinib (commonly known as Tarceva).

There were just a few little problems. First, Tarceva—the subject of expansive molecular analyses—was increasingly identified as a treatment of choice for Asian, nonsmoking females. Rick, our Caucasian male with a history of smoking and substance abuse, didn't exactly fit the profile. Second, the drug cost several thousand dollars per month.

Contrary to every expectation, Rick's disease disappeared. The toxicities, principally skin rash and some early lung symptoms, became more tolerable. Rick returned to his normal activities and would visit me occasionally on his motorcycle for follow-ups.

A year later, now two years on hospice, Rick's follow-up PET/CT revealed the persistence of uptake (activity possibly reflective of persistent cancer) along the surface of the lung where he had had the original biopsy. The findings were in the exact same location as the prior biopsy. Biopsies often leave residual scars, which light up on PET scan. But it was in this area that Rick experienced persistent pain. The VA advised him to increase his pain medications or undergo surgery to kill the nerve bundle sending the pain signals.

I was troubled by the pain Rick was experiencing, but I could not say with certainty whether this was scar tissue or recurrent disease. We decided to have interventional radiology conduct core biopsies under guidance to resolve the question. To our delight the findings were benign. "Talc granuloma" read the pathology report describing the microscopic appearance of the scar associated with talcum powder used by the surgeon to seal the section after the original November 2005 biopsy.

Relieved, Rick continued his busy schedule.

Another year passed and the pain persisted. Rick returned to Cedars-Sinai for another opinion and met with skilled thoracic surgeon Dr. Robert McKenna Jr., who carefully reviewed the records and Rick's most recent PET/CT scan. He then summoned Rick and his girlfriend Jennifer into his office where, peering over his large mahogany desk, he said, "You are riddled with cancer."

"What?" said Rick dumbfounded.

Dr. McKenna carefully explained that the areas surrounding the lungs were filled with cancerous lesions. Rick asked, "What's the next step?"

"We'll have to get another biopsy."

Rick agreed to undergo a thoracotomy. It was decided that the area of the pleural surface, recognized by multiple PET/CT scans and previously found at the time of biopsy to be a talc granuloma, needed to be resected. With bated breath, we awaited the findings, which upon pathological review proved to be—talc granuloma.

Another year later, now four years on hospice, Rick's PET scan again revealed an area of uptake along the left chest wall. By now, Rick had gained weight, was working full time, and all of his blood tests were normal. Concerned by the cystic area on the CT scan, along the left lung surface, Dr. Shuman and I agreed that a biopsy was needed. Though we stood at the ready to conduct an additional analysis if needed, we realized following careful histological review of the tissue removed that you never give chemotherapy to treat a talc granuloma.

Rick Carroll remains well and free of disease and, as I now write this, it's approaching six years since we met. He is but one example of how we believe patients can outlive cancer. Indeed, Rick is also living proof that you can outlive hospice.

1 2

East Meets West

O ne evening in early 1985, during my hematology fellowship at Scripps Clinic in La Jolla, California, I joined my friend and colleague Sheldon S. Hendler, PhD, MD, author, scientist, and professor of biochemistry, at his home for dinner. There, I was introduced to Dr. Alan Kapuler. Alan had received his PhD in molecular biochemistry from the Rockefeller University and completed his postdoctoral work at the Rothschild Institute in Paris, France. He then joined the faculty at the University of Connecticut in Storrs.

During this time he had made discoveries that, in retrospect, have changed the way we think about human biology. On this particular evening, Alan was suffering from a respiratory infection and treating himself with an herbal remedy that he had prepared. As we discussed the medicinal value of the herbs he had chosen in the preparation of his potion, it became evident to me that his knowledge of plant biology was nothing less than extraordinary.

By the time we met, Alan had long since left his university post, after coming to blows with his academic peers, and had traveled west to establish an organic, planetary gene-pool resource and service—that is, a hippie seed company in Oregon.

Alan, a product of the sixties, had a unique way of "turning on and dropping out." His way was to apply his manifest skills in genomics to the study of plant biodiversity and evolutionary genetics.

Using his knowledge, Alan realized he could conserve species that were at risk of extinction while developing new ones that had never been seen before. Using kinship maps (measures of plant species relationships), he could recognize how seemingly unrelated plants could be crossbred to provide ears of corn rich in purple anthocyanins (sought after for their antioxidant properties in fruits like blueberries and grapes), as well as tomatoes with large amounts of the psychologically uplifting neurotransmitter GABA (gamma amino butyric acid).

After our initial introduction, I had little contact with Alan until I received a call several years later. Alan had been diagnosed with advanced stage non-Hodgkin B-cell lymphoma. With his broad knowledge of nucleotide biochemistry (DNA and RNA), he had grave misgivings about conventional (cytotoxic) chemotherapy drugs. Nonetheless, he did agree to submit a portion of a lymph node biopsy to my laboratory for analysis. The following week with the pathology report in hand (B-cell, mixed, intermediate grade, Stage IV non-Hodgkin lymphoma), I recommended a modification of a standard chemotherapy combination (C-MOPP) based upon our laboratory findings.

"Are you kidding?" he responded with dismay. "Do you have any idea what those chemotherapy drugs do to your chromosomes?"

"Yes," I responded. "That's why they work."

"Not for me," he replied. And flatly refused the recommended chemotherapy.

Brainiac that he was, Alan undertook a thorough study of his options. He settled upon the teachings of Michio Kushi and macrobiotics, after his mother-in-law, Elma, gave him a copy of Aveline Kushi's book *Introduction to Macrobiotic Cooking*. What followed was a complete makeover of Alan's life. He eliminated caffeine, sugar, meat, and cigarettes (as well as his beloved marijuana). He adopted the yin/yang principles, balancing his every intake. He was going to beat his lymphoma naturally. I was mortified. Alan was going to die. I knew I could help him, unlike some of the patients I saw, maybe cure him, and he was going to refuse my care. Alan was going to die on my watch.

No amount of arguing on my part would convince him. And so, I watched and waited, expecting the phone to ring with his wife, Linda, on the other end, begging me to initiate treatment. But the call never came. Alan got better. His lymph nodes got smaller, his symptoms resolved, he gained weight, and he returned to normal activities—for three and a half years.

So remarkable was his saga that he caught the attention of Andrew Weil, MD, who included Alan in chapter 3, pages 54–58 in his book *Spontaneous Healing*. That was enough for me. I went out and bought every Michio Kushi book I could find. I began to attend naturopathic conferences, even speaking at a few. Needless to say, I was extremely impressed by this remarkable remission.

As Alan approached more than three years of well-being, the wheels began to fall off. The lymph nodes grew, he began to lose weight, and his lymphoma was clearly on the march. I saw him in clinical follow-up and recommended a biopsy to reevaluate his chemotherapeutic options. He declined and traveled to the Bio-Medical Center in Tijuana, Mexico, where he undertook additional efforts with the Hoxsey formula (a natural combination of herbs, with potassium iodide) and a variety of immune augmentative therapies, which put the lymphoma in remission for another three years.

Four years later, he returned to my office for a consultation. I examined him and noted palpable lymph nodes in the area just below the left neck. He explained that they had been growing slowly and that he had more symptoms of fever and weight loss. I urged him to allow me to rebiopsy the site, but he declined. He wanted to avoid conventional chemotherapeutics at all costs. I was deeply concerned that the costs would be dearer than he might imagine.

Two months later, Alan again returned. By now, the lymphoma was consuming him. Alan had lymph nodes in places other people didn't have places. Running down his anterior chest and along his abdomen were small nodules filled with malignant lymphocytes that protruded like nipples on a dog. He had lumps in his groin, armpits, and neck. He even had lymph nodes on his elbows. More concerning, his x-ray revealed a complete replacement of the chest cavity with fluid, causing a "white out" of the image on the film. Alan was dying, and this time he knew it.

The laboratory assay results provided an interesting opportunity. Based upon work I had done several years earlier, I included in the laboratory analysis the combination of a purine analog and an alkylating agent. Going back to my first days at Scripps Clinic, a closely related combination (nitrogen mustard plus 2CDA) had revealed one of the best profiles of any combination I had ever tested (Nagourney 1993). Alan fit the profile perfectly. I admitted him to the hospital immediately. I still recall the thoracentesis (fluid removal from the chest) that I conducted the day of his admission. I removed more fluid from his chest than I have ever removed from any other patient before or since—four liters.

Alan detested the idea of chemotherapy. Everything about it rubbed him the wrong way. But he was comforted to know that the drugs I selected were, in my estimation, exactly right for him. What was interesting was that this particular combination was not generally used for this type of lymphoma (I would probably go so far as to say, *never*). Ironically, the fact that we were not adhering to generally accepted guidelines probably comforted him.

I explained that should the treatment actually prove effective, the silver lining would be the lack of hair loss associated with chemotherapy. If all went well, Alan would preserve his long, flowing beard and Sikh-like hair coiled up under a woven cap that he wore like a Rastafarian. The first week was very tough. Alan was desperately ill and the chemotherapy's side effects didn't sit well with him. Almost immediately, however, the lymph nodes began to shrink. He stopped being in intense pain and the fluid in the chest didn't re-accumulate. By the end of the second week, he was feeling reasonably well and returned to La Jolla to stay with our mutual friend Dr. Hendler, while he awaited the initiation of cycle two. With each successive treatment (given every three weeks) his condition improved. By the end of the sixth cycle, he was well and free of disease by all radiographic and biochemical parameters.

Alan returned to his normal life and has sent me many patients over the years. Interestingly, he was never exposed to the more toxic classes of drugs associated with cardiac risks and neurological toxicities. Instead, he enjoyed the benefit of a relatively simple two-drug combination while avoiding many of the toxicities associated with lymphoma treatment.

At the tenth year—almost to the day—Alan presented with flank pain suggestive of a kidney stone. A more formal workup revealed, by PET scan, evidence of abnormal lymph nodes in the retroperitoneal space (the anatomic area lying behind the abdominal organs running from diaphragm to pelvis). The biopsy confirmed non-Hodgkin B-cell lymphoma similar to the diagnosis ten years earlier. This time, the laboratory findings recommended bendamustine. This newly available drug has a chemical structure that combines the mustard alkylator and purine analog backbones—highly reminiscent of the combination we'd used a decade earlier.

Alan returned to Oregon where an accomplished German-trained medical oncologist, Dieter Morich, MD, kindly offered to administer the schedule outlined and, at the time that I write this book, he has finished his treatment and is again in complete remission.

I am a great believer that physicians can learn from their patients. Alan's excellent and durable response to a natural therapy program of his own design was a case in point. Despite my classical training in allopathic medicine, interest and study of pharmacology, and background in chemistry, I had never seriously considered the merit of naturopathy. That is, not until Alan's lymph node melted away and he returned to a normal life using little more than soy miso, green tea, organic foods, and lifestyle adjustments.

Alan is living proof that there is much more to the study of cancer and human biology than chemotherapy.

Alan also enabled me to prove that a durable and complete remission could be achieved without the toxicity of standard "CHOP" chemotherapy. His success enabled me to apply this double regimen in many patients over the years. This same combination has become the gold standard for low-grade lymphoma and chronic lymphocytic leukemia today.

A final lesson from Alan was the fact that he remained as sensitive as he had been in the beginning. His excellent response again enabled him to avoid the toxicity of a more aggressive regimen. I am pleased that Alan has done so well. His Peace Seeds repository of plant species and brilliance (as well as his friendship) make him a resource the world could ill afford to lose.

Garlic, Wine, Chocolate, and More

My experience with Alan Kapuler had a profound effect upon me. The certainty that nontraditional medicine had no merit melted away as I examined Alan's unequivocal, irrefutable response to little more than diet and lifestyle changes. What, after all, was in the miso, honey, whole grains, green vegetables, berries, and green tea that could provide such an outcome?

Having purchased Michio Kushi's many books on macrobiotics, I examined the precepts of locally grown vegetables and balancing yin with yang. I attended conferences on complementary medicine and took my patients' suggestions that their diet, yoga, Qigong, acupressure, acupuncture, aromatherapy, and meditation did indeed influence their outcomes. It was about this time that my colleague Dr. Hendler, MD, PhD, was asked by Mary Ann Liebert to edit a new journal dedicated to this field of investigation. The *Journal of Medicinal Food* (*JMF*) was launched in the summer of 1998, and I was invited to join the editorial board. Indeed, I was invited to write the lead article for the inaugural issue.

THE STINKING ROSE AND OTHER DELIGHTS

I chose garlic as my topic. As the publication date drew closer, I found myself drowning in garlic publications. Little did I realize at the time I accepted the offer that there were more than 1,300 peer-reviewed publications on the topic of garlic as a medicinal food. Compulsive overachiever that I am, I did my best to read every one. Night after night, I worked into the wee hours compiling, reviewing, editing, rewriting, and re-reviewing the topic. Finally, with almost 300 references excerpted from the literature, my treatise on garlic was published.

The journal became a window on the chemistry of foodstuffs, spices, and biological actives. I found myself reviewing manuscripts on rose extracts, chocolate, and red wine, and writing editorials on genetically modified organisms and their influence on biodiversity.

With my newfound expertise I began to lecture on the topics that I encountered in the journal. One of my most popular and best-received lectures, one that I have given several times, is entitled "Garlic, Wine, and Chocolate." For obvious reasons, it's a popular presentation.

I begin my lecture by reminding the audience that, however nuanced the human experience, our existence as biological entities reflects little more than the transfer of two electrons from molecular oxygen to water. As such, success in life reflects efficient electron management. After all, life on earth evolved in an environment fraught with free radical activity, initiated by the release into the atmosphere of molecular oxygen (O_2) by primordial photosynthetic blue-green algae. Our diets contain substances that offer protection against oxidative damage; some foods can be particularly beneficial.

Garlic, wine, and chocolate all contain polyphenols, flavonoids, and thiols (sulfur-containing chemicals) capable of detoxifying chemical reactants. Garlic is an excellent source of thiols, including thiosulfinates and allyl sulfides, while wine and chocolate are rich with phenolics, anthocyanins, and stilbenes.

The botany of garlic places it as a member of the lily family. *Allium sativa* (garlic) is a member of a group that includes onions, leeks, shallots, and chives. According to Alphonse De Candolle (*The Origin of Cultivated Plants,* 1908), garlic came from the Kirgiz region of Siberia more than 6,000 years ago, and from there was brought to Asia Minor, India, China, and finally Europe and the New World. Of the more than two million metric tons produced each year, China produces and consumes the most, with the United States a distant sixth in production and consumption. Gilroy, California, dubbed "the garlic capital of the United States," was once noted by humorist Will Rogers to be "the only town in America where you can marinate a steak by hanging it on a clothesline."

Garlic's role in cancer has been the subject of many studies. When the incidence of gastric cancer in two counties in the Shandong province of China was compared, the people of Gangshang, who consumed 20 grams per day, had one-thirteenth the incidence of cancer when compared to people of the neighboring Qixia district who ate only one gram per day (Mei 1982). Case-controlled studies in Italy found similar benefits, as did American studies that examined colon cancer in women in the Midwest.

There are many suggested mechanisms by which garlic may influence carcinogenesis, including a direct interaction with toxins, as well as the induction of detoxifying enzymes. Garlic has many other properties of interest, including the capacity to lower cholesterol and protect against infection. My belief in garlic as a medicinal is well established by our household's monthly consumption of between two and three liters of peeled cloves.

I then turn to *Vitis vinifera*—the grape from which wine is produced. Following fermentation, grapes provide hundreds of varieties of wine that have been produced for millennia. The phenols in red wine include simple phenols like gallic acid, as well as the stilbenes (for example, resveratrol), flavonoids (for example, quercetin), and anthocyanins. Resveratrol, a compound that has garnered significant attention in recent years, has many biological properties, including gene regulation and inhibition of the estrogen receptor. A study of Spanish red wines found an average of 18.8 mg of resveratrol per liter (Moreno-Labanda 2004). The most abundant flavonoids in red wine are the catechins.

The polyphenols of red wine have antioxidant properties, dilate blood vessels (via nitric oxide production), and can inhibit blood clotting. They can also reduce inflammation. Based upon these properties, red wine has been associated with a decline in prostate cancer and appears superior to other alcoholic beverages in this regard.

My final discussion in these lectures focuses on chocolate—the extract of *Theobroma cacao*. Originating in Mayan and Aztec cultures, xocolatl (as it was known) was harvested, fermented, dried, and roasted to produce cocoa mass—a mixture of cocoa butter and cocoa solid. Brought to Europe by Columbus in 1502, chocolate was considered a luxury, available only to the wealthy.

The composition of chocolate reveals 54 percent cocoa butter, 11 percent protein, up to 10 percent fiber, another 10 percent organic acids, with a small amount of theobromine and caffeine. It is the polyphenolic content of chocolate, constituting 12 to 18 percent of the dry weight, that provides some of its most healthful features. Not surprisingly, dark chocolate, 59 percent cocoa solid, is the healthiest.

Sophisticated analyses of chocolate's properties have revealed interesting findings—among them, the inhibition of the cancer-promoting enzyme telomerase, induction of apoptosis, and decrease of NF-kB (a potent mediator of inflammation). It has long been known that inflammation is closely associated with cancer. Chocolate's anti-inflammatory properties may be important in cancer prevention.

Strikingly, a comparison of chocolate, wine, and green tea favored chocolate for phenolic and flavonoid content, clearly supporting the role of chocolate as a medicinal food. One of the curiosities of chocolate is its loyal following among those who call themselves "chocoholics." While the stimulatory effect of the methylxanthines like caffeine may be responsible, this addiction may also be attributed to a trace compound known as anandamide. This compound binds to the same receptors that are triggered by the cannabinoids found in marijuana, resulting in what has been described as chocolate bliss. In the literature, anandamide has been said to be "more than a food, less than a drug." It wasn't until 1996 that we recognized chocolate to be a source of anandamide. Interestingly, there are no other known foodstuffs that contain this compound.

My reasons for lecturing on these topics are numerous. First, the provision of red wine, my own garlic dressing recipe, and dark chocolate desserts are a big hit with the audience. Second, I want to educate people on the bona fide health benefits of these simple foodstuffs. I particularly like promoting garlic, as it is a food that I consume in great quantities.

Finally, I want to introduce the public to the very real, very scientific basis of diet as an adjunct to health. Numerous studies have suggested that dietary supplements in and of themselves may not only fail to provide healthful benefits, but may actually be deleterious. The CARET Study (Omenn 1996), conducted in Northern Europe, that provided cigarette smokers with beta-carotene (naturally found in fruit and vegetables) supplementation resulted in a significant increase in cancer deaths. More recently, the SELECT study (Lippman 2009) that administered vitamin E, with or without selenium, to men at risk for prostate cancer has recently revealed a 17 percent increase in prostate cancer for the men who consumed vitamin E alone.

What these and related studies may actually be telling us is that it is not the chemical activity that provides the benefit, but the foodstuffs that contain them. It is in this light that my lecture on garlic, wine, and chocolate promotes healthy diet over dietary supplements as the preferred lifestyle adjustment.

OTHER HEALTHY FOOD POSSIBILITIES

In addition to these investigations, I conducted a clinical trial of the citrus fruit extract limonene, found in the zest of oranges and lemons. When I combined limonene with the cholesterol-lowering drug Zocor (simvastatin), I observed objective responses in several cancer patients, including measurable changes in chest x-ray and declines in prostate-specific antigens (PSA).

I was later intrigued by a manuscript I reviewed for the *Journal of Medicinal Food*, which described the healthful effects of the chemicals extracted from the entire orange peel, not just the zest, the source of the limonene. As I considered the findings surrounding whole orange peel, I was reminded of an article authored by Linus Pauling with the Scottish surgeon Ewan Cameron, published in the 1980s in the *New England Journal of Medicine*. This study of vitamin C supplementation for cancer patients failed to establish the benefit. Might we now reexamine that study and realize that Pauling's premise (the benefits of vitamin C supplementation) may, indeed, have been correct. But it was the source of vitamin C—citrus fruits—that contributed the benefit, not just the chemical ascorbic acid (vitamin C). Had I used whole orange peel, might I have seen even better responses than those observed with the extract in my study?

Over and over again, it seems we outsmart ourselves. Our penchant to reduce biology to its constituent components rather than accepting its complexity has led us down blind alleys more than once. I, for one, enjoy a glass of red wine, consume dark chocolate, and enjoy garlic in astonishing quantities.

14

Treatable Cancers Should Be Treated Correctly

Conventional wisdom in oncology would suggest that patient outcomes are predicated upon prognostic categories. That is, patients with drug-sensitive diseases like leukemia and lymphoma do better than patients with drug-resistant diseases like lung cancer and melanoma. Within each category are subsets designated by grade (degree of atypia), stage (extent of spread), and a growing panoply of immunohistochemical and molecular markers like HER2, EGFR, ER, PR, and more.

These are the cornerstones of oncologic prognostication. *Prognosis*, from the Greek, means "to know before." In this instance, the oncologist knows how the patient is likely to do before he or she ever meets them. That's because prognostic factors are general categorizations. An obvious example being that males are much more likely to get prostate cancer than females, while females are much more likely to get ovarian cancer than males. This is because men don't have ovaries and women don't have prostates. Going in, the doctor has a general sense of what to expect. But that's the problem. It's a very general sense.

Once we move from generic categorization to individual patient selection, these and related factors break the sound barrier and become predictive factors.

Prediction, from the Latin, means "to say before." Predictive factors are those determinats that tell you, on an individual patient basis, what is likely to happen. Those patients in this chapter clearly define that a bad prognosis can be overcome by a good prediction. While high-grade breast cancer and metastatic pancreatic cancer fall into the worst prognostic groups, sensitivity to available therapies trumps all.

INGRID INSISTS ON AN ASSAY

Ingrid Ottesen, a strapping sixty-nine-year-old Norwegian woman who came to my office in September 1997, had estrogen receptor (ER)–positive breast cancer. That was the good news. The finding of estrogen positivity is associated with better outcomes and response to simple medications like Tamoxifen. It wasn't until after her surgery that I discovered the bad news: thirteen positive lymph nodes. Patients with breast cancer whose disease has spread to the lymph nodes (lymph node–positive disease) are candidates for chemotherapy. Those with one to three positive lymph nodes do better than those with four or more. There's a special name for those with more than ten positive lymph nodes—dead.

It seems that patients whose cancers spread so rapidly that they invade and fill up the axilla (armpit) with cancer-containing lymph nodes, virtually all go on to progress and die. In one large clinical trial, the Taxotere-based chemotherapy TAC (Taxotere plus Adriamycin plus Cytoxan) that bested the control arm of FAC (5-FU plus Adriamycin plus Cytoxan) had little impact on patients with more than ten positive lymph nodes with similar survivals, regardless of which arm of the study they went on (Martin 2005).

This was the situation that Ingrid would soon find herself in. However, on this September afternoon, as we met for the first time, neither she nor I had any idea what lay ahead.

After an initial biopsy conducted in July 1997 confirmed Ingrid's diagnosis, she obtained an opinion from prominent surgeon Melvin J. Silverstein, MD, at the University of Southern California. He recommended a right mastectomy. With the mass in the right breast and the palpable lymph node in the right armpit, Ingrid appeared to be a good candidate for this treatment option. After review at the tumor board, based upon the multicentric disease (involving many areas within the breast) and the relatively high-grade tumor features (scored 7 out of 9 on a scale of 1–9, 9 being worst), the recommendation was to proceed with the mastectomy. It appeared to me that the patient could undergo conventional chemo and hormonal therapies and would not require any further evaluation from my laboratory or me. I still remember dissuading the patient from submitting tissue to my laboratory following surgery, inasmuch as I anticipated that she would undergo her mastectomy and be referred to one of the many capable medical oncologists in the community.

Despite my recommendation to forgo assay analysis, Ingrid—in her own wisdom—insisted that her surgeon submit a portion of her tumor. At the time of surgery, the findings were not good. The pathologist found a 2.5 centimeter, high-grade infiltrating ductal carcinoma that was ER positive, progesterone receptor (PR) negative and, more worrisome, human epidermal growth factor receptor 2 (HER2) positive. (HER2 is a protein that encourages the growth of cancer cells, and HER2-positive breast cancers are often more aggressive with a tendency to involve lymph nodes and spread rapidly to distant sites.) However, this paled in comparison to the finding of thirteen lymph nodes positive for metastatic disease.

Several days later, as I completed my laboratory analyses, Ingrid's pathology report arrived. With thirteen positive lymph nodes, I knew then that Ingrid had made the right choice.

Our lab results, in retrospect, presaged later developments and the concept that HER2-positive tumors were better candidates for Adriamycin-based therapy. (Subsequent work by Dennis Slamon, MD, PhD, confirmed an association between the HER2 gene and the topoisomerase 2A gene, the latter being the target for Adriamycin. As such, a subset of HER2 patients are hypersensitive to

Adriamycin.) With these results in hand, we recommended a dose-dense—high doses, repeated frequently—Cytoxan plus Adriamycin combination.

The laboratory analysis offered an additional insight. Consistent with our developing use of cisplatin plus gemcitabine in breast cancer (Nagourney 2000), Ingrid revealed a highly favorable profile for this novel doublet. As I pondered the lethality of thirteen positive lymph nodes, I recommended a post–Cytoxan plus Adriamycin reinforcement of cisplatin plus gemcitabine, something that today would be considered aggressive; in 1997 it was unheard of.

Ingrid tolerated the treatment well, but suffered what I would have to describe as a remarkable degree of alopecia. I believe every hair on her body fell off—from scalp to eyebrows and eyelashes and everywhere else, I presume. She recovered well and tolerated the second-line therapy of cisplatin plus gemcitabine extremely well. In 1997, the finding of HER2 overexpression was little more than an adverse prognostic finding—that is, patients with HER2-positive tumors tended to do worse. The antibody Herceptin, directed against HER2-positive tumors, was not yet available and at this time no one would ever imagine using it in the postoperative setting.

Recognizing the gravity of Ingrid's diagnosis, I followed her every three months and waited for the other shoe to drop.

But it didn't. Not the first year or the second, or the fifth or the tenth. Ingrid Ottesen had dodged a nuclear weapon. Her cancer was biologically programmed to metastasize and recur—high-grade, large, multicentric, HER2 positive, and with thirteen positive lymph nodes. Nobody survived this kind of cancer—nobody, that is, except Ingrid.

Year by year, Ingrid would return for follow-up. She knit my children sweaters and matching hats out of blue-and-white wool with traditional Norwegian snowflake designs. She brought me calendars, cheese slicers, souvenir spoons, and other gifts from her yearly travels to Norway. She brought her dogs, her friends, and her occasional complaints of aches and pains, but never once did she bring me any evidence of recurrent cancer.

What was it about Ingrid or another patient, Evelyn Salvador, a charming fifty-five-year-old Filipino female with an almost identical presentation for whom I provided an almost identical therapy? Why did they survive? For that matter, why does anyone survive?

Most doctors would respond, "It's their biology." And in a way, I would agree. For these doctors, the good outcomes of these two patients were the chance event of patients receiving the right treatments for their biology.

For me, however, there was nothing random about it. Ingrid had the right biology, and I knew it going in. Her good outcome wasn't an accident; it was a function of her tumor's exquisite sensitivity to alkylating agents, anthracyclines, and the combination of cisplatin plus gemcitabine that we identified in the laboratory that first day. Ingrid was destined to respond to that combination—and I knew it.

Now, fourteen years later, I better understand what I learned about Ingrid that day. Her cancer cells had forgotten how to die. But our laboratory findings instructed us that Cytoxan, Adriamycin, and cisplatin plus gemcitabine would remind them of their own mortality. Today, following the introduction of Herceptin, good outcomes in HER2-positive patients are more common. But in 1997, the pre-Herceptin era, Ingrid's good outcome stands as a monument to laboratory-directed therapy.

Now an octogenarian, Ingrid has recently designed and is preparing for production of a new type of articulated gurney for the transport of patients in hospitals. A physical therapist by training, accomplished athlete, and unstoppable force of nature, this Norwegian she-wolf might just live to market a new and important device for the management of injured patients and those in need of physical therapy—fourteen years after she was handed a death sentence.

ANOTHER DEADLY DIAGNOSIS TURNED AWAY

There are two kinds of patients with cancer of the pancreas: those who can be treated and those who can't. Unfortunately, no one has ever taken the time to figure out who's who. When a patient is diagnosed with pancreatic cancer, they're provided statistics that could not be grimmer. Few, if any, are good candidates for surgery. Even for those who do qualify for the highly aggressive Whipple procedure—removal of the distal portion of the stomach, gallbladder, cystic and bile ducts, the head of the pancreas, duodenum, proximal jejunum, and regional lymph nodes—cancer almost invariably recurs. For those who present with metastatic disease, the median survival is a paltry four to six months.

When Steve Lockwood presented to his physician with a several-month history of abdominal pain, he received nonsteroidal anti-inflammatory drugs without benefit. The findings of anemia led to an ultrasound and then a CT scan. The news could hardly have been worse. A 5 cm x 4 cm x 3 cm mass in the tail of the pancreas was encasing the splenic vein. The abdominal cavity was awash in cancer cells and his liver was nearly completely replaced by tumor. A CT-guided biopsy confirmed the worst. Steve met with a qualified medical oncologist in Torrance, California, and then sought second opinions at UCLA and the City of Hope. All delivered the same dismal news. When his wife, a registered nurse, brought Steve to see me, he was in a steep downward spiral.

He was in extraordinary pain, with unrelenting nausea and vomiting. He was losing weight and his tumor markers were doubling by the week, now well into the thousands (normal is zero to thirty). Steve seemed so terribly ill, I wondered whether I could help him at all. But I knew no one else could. So, I arranged for an open surgical biopsy the next day.

Within a week, I had the results of our laboratory analysis. Steve was a slam dunk for a three-drug combination that I had used extensively in the past. We started treatment immediately. Despite my confidence that I'd selected the right drugs, and the speed with which treatment began, his condition continued to deteriorate. His tumor markers rose unabated, now cresting near 6,000. The nausea and pain were unbearable. Indeed, I brought him into the infusion center every day for IV hydration to prevent him from becoming clinically dehydrated. Despite his size (six feet) and build (muscular) I couldn't imagine where he was putting two liters of fluid each day.

With the first two-week cycle of therapy under our belt, I brought Steve back for his first follow-up visit. He felt a little better. Not a lot, mind you, not much at all, but enough to say that he thought it might be working. I had no objective evidence to go on other than my certainty that the treatment was right for him. We elected to do another round.

By the sixth week, he *was* better, much better. Better in every way. He stopped his pain medications and started eating. He even felt hungry.

He still needed hydration, but only around the days of treatment. The rest of the time he felt well. Best of all, his tumor markers stopped rising and actually began falling.

Steve's next cycle was a turning point. He felt well, had gained a significant amount of weight, and was eating a regular diet. He was tolerating the treatment better and looked good. By cycle four, Steven was still better. He had good color, had maintained his weight, and was leading an active and normal lifestyle.

As we met, prior to his fifth cycle of treatment, he complained of swelling in his leg. I examined him and made a clinical diagnosis of deep venous thrombosis (DVT) of the lower extremity. The complication of DVT, also known as phlebitis, is well known to those of us who treat pancreatic cancer. This finding, originally described by Armand Trousseau in the 1860s (now known as Trousseau's sign), reflects the tendency of patients with mucinous adenocarcinomas to form blood clots. This clotting tendency, known as hypercoagulability, is a worrisome sign as it often heralds progression of the disease.

I was crestfallen. My patient appeared to be progressing, despite my expectations to the contrary. As I discussed the finding and its implications with the patient, raising my concerns, his wife cajoled him to come clean. As it turns out, Steve was feeling so good that he spent the entire weekend horseback riding. Not surprisingly, the chronic pressure of the saddle had caused the blood clot, not progression of his disease. I was pleased and a little amused. From now on, I would need to remember to tell all my patients with metastatic pancreatic cancer to limit their horseback riding to only six hours a day!

To confirm our success we conducted a PET/CT scan. The scan showed dramatic improvement, with only faint residual disease in the area of the pancreas. The tumor markers were now normal. Steve was one of those unusual pancreatic cancer patients who did well, very well.

At this point the questions were "how much therapy" and "for how long?"

We were at six cycles and I recommended eight. By early 2011, with normal PET/CT scans, normal CA 19-9, normal CEA, and normal liver function tests, there was no disease to be found. But I knew it probably wasn't gone for good.

Our discussions then focused on my personal bias for maintenance therapies. The concept of continuous treatments (maintenance) went in and out of favor in the medical literature, never gaining wide appeal except in pediatric leukemia populations. In retrospect, the failure of maintenance therapy to catch on in adult patients most likely represents the random selection of drug treatments, rarity of complete remission, and, as a result, the diminishing returns associated with additional therapy.

Bad drugs don't work no matter how long you give them. Yet, good drugs continue to work indefinitely. How this simple concept has continued to elude medical oncologists is, in part, the reason I write this book.

It was decided. Steve would go on a maintenance schedule one week out of three—the same drugs, the same doses, just less frequently. He and his wife celebrated their sixteen-year anniversary on March 11, 2011. That happened to be the same day that he was to start a round of therapy. When I offered to postpone the treatment, his wife, Joan, told me she couldn't think of a better way to celebrate.

As of this writing, in August 2012, Steve remains in complete remission approaching two and one-half years. As remarkable as his case may be, he is one of many patients with metastatic pancreatic cancer who have outlived expectations by years, and in one case, by more than a decade.

15

When All Else Fails

"**D**r. Nagourney, there's a physician from Cincinnati on the telephone who would like to speak to you about his wife," said Shari Burt, director of patient/physician relations at Rational Therapeutics.

As I always make every effort to speak with referring physicians, I took the call in my office. "This is Thomas Panke," said the man on the other end of the phone. There was a tone of desperation and tension in his voice. "I'd like to talk to you about my wife." I sat and listened intently as he described the difficulties that he and his wife had encountered since her first diagnosis with advanced ovarian cancer.

Tom explained, "On July 6, 1999, my wife, Liz, underwent TAH-BSO (total abdominal hysterectomy and bilateral oophorectomy—the standard surgical procedure for advanced ovarian cancer) for Stage IIIC (extensive) ovarian carcinoma at Bethesda North Hospital in Cincinnati. As soon as she recovered, she began chemotherapy with carboplatin plus Taxol. After two cycles, the disease was rapidly progressing. Her medical oncologist, Peter Ruehlman, MD, immediately changed her to second-line therapy with topotecan. Within two cycles of topotecan and all of the associated toxicities, her disease raged forward and was now producing four liters of abdominal ascites fluid every week."

As we spoke, it became evident that this was a highly sophisticated physician with an extraordinary grasp of our work. When I inquired, he explained that he was the medical director of Pathology Services of the TriHealth System, the largest healthcare system in the Cincinnati area.

At their last meeting, Dr. Ruehlman told Liz to "get her affairs in order." He then took Tom aside and told him that she would not see Christmas. It was October 21, 1999, Elizabeth Panke had platinum-resistant ovarian cancer, and she was preparing to die.

Born in Poland and educated in the United States, Liz had obtained her medical degree and PhD, with training in pathology. She went on to establish a successful molecular genetics corporation, Genetica, in Cincinnati, and had faced adversity many times in her life. Neither Liz nor her husband, Tom—who doted on her— was willing to give up. Instead, they took a leave of absence and traveled to every major medical institution with expertise in the management of advanced ovarian cancer in the United States. From the Cleveland Clinic to the University of Indiana, Indianapolis; from Memorial Sloan-Kettering in New York to M.D. Anderson in Texas; from the University of California, Davis, to Ohio State University, Columbus; and finally to my alma mater, the University of California, Irvine. No one, but no one, had an answer.

Each physician explained that "platinum-resistant" ovarian cancer that had failed salvage therapy was incurable. More disturbing was the fact that the suggestions provided by the physicians from each of these well-respected institutions didn't agree. When there is no right answer to a question, there are always many wrong answers. In retrospect, the most disturbing fact was that not a single physician in any one of these facilities ever mentioned that laboratory tests existed that could provide guidance for the selection of therapy.

Left to their own devices, Tom and Liz turned to the Internet for answers. They learned of a company in Southern California that offered a lab test called the EDR analysis. The company, Oncotech, provided a service designed to "eliminate" inactive drugs by measuring extreme drug resistance (EDR)—a finding that the company purported would confirm a near-zero likelihood of response when identified for a given drug. However accurate the EDR test might or might not have been in eliminating drugs, it did not, in fact it *could* not, identify active drugs. As a co-founder of Oncotech, I knew only too well the limitations of the EDR method. In fact, it was those limitations that ultimately led to my departure from the company.

This nuance was lost to the desperate Pankes who submitted a liter of fluid to Oncotech hoping that an active drug would be identified.

Days later, still scouring the Internet, they came across a reference to me. The phone call was placed, and I was now sitting in my office attempting to comfort an obviously desperate and loving husband, who was confronting the unavoidable death of his cherished wife.

"Can you help my wife?" he asked. "We've just sent a sample to Oncotech."

"Oh dear," I muttered without being able to repress my reflexive response. I was only too familiar with Oncotech's inability to select active drugs. I then asked, "Has she received any recent therapy?"

"No," replied Tom.

"Is there still fluid?"

"Ample," he replied.

"Could you send me a sample?" I asked.

"Absolutely," he responded.

I told him that I would do everything I could to help and would provide my results within seven days. I further explained that my ability to conduct the analysis was dependent on an adequate sample, that it remain alive during the period of the test, that she be sensitive to some drug or combination, and that even my best attempts to find an active drug would only improve her odds, not guarantee an outcome. I explained that the test required 72 to 96 hours during which time the isolated tumor cells would be exposed to the drugs and combinations of interest. After the analyses were completed, calculations conducted, and results compared with our ovarian cancer database, I promised I would follow up as soon as possible. We agreed to be in touch and I hung up.

The following morning, November 8, 1999, the sample arrived.

Every day, Tom Panke called me and asked if the results were ready. And every day I told him it took 72 to 96 hours, the same thing I had told him the day before. In the interim, the Oncotech assay, submitted the week before mine, was completed. Ironically, Oncotech had recommended carboplatin, Taxol, and topotecan, the exact three drugs Liz had just failed. The results weren't wrong (that is, *extreme* resistance had not been identified); they just weren't helpful. Patients in Liz's situation don't need help eliminating drugs; they need help finding active drugs. Oncotech's assay couldn't find active drugs.

On the fourth day, Tom called. I said that we would be taking the lab analysis down and would call him with the result.

That evening, I worked late. The laboratory technicians had completed the day's work and Liz's assay awaited final review. I sat with my senior medical technician at the double-headed microscope and scored the assay's results. Not surprisingly, most of the drugs were inactive. But one combination killed every cell at every concentration. The combination was cisplatin plus gemcitabine, our ace in the hole.

It so happened that this was a combination I had been developing for more than five years, one that had shown extraordinary promise in ovarian and breast cancers, as well as other disease types. Not yet in the published literature, the combination was only beginning to be used and was not considered a treatment for ovarian cancer patients. But I knew beyond a shadow of a doubt that this was the treatment for Liz.

This combination of two drugs was among our most important proof-of-concept for the value of laboratory-directed therapy. It works for reasons that had escaped most oncologists. With the luxury of our laboratory platform as our testing ground, we developed this doublet from scratch.

If you ask any oncologist, he or she will tell you that patients who that have failed platinum-based therapy have a vanishingly small chance of responding to this drug ever again. In fact, doctors will simply refuse to give it. In point of fact, resistance to cisplatin, or its closely related relative carboplatin, proves to be among the worst factors for the management of advanced ovarian cancer. Indeed, clinical protocols define treatment candidates as "platin sensitive" and "platin resistant," as separate and distinct categories of disease.

Using our laboratory model in ovarian cancer patients, we found something quite extraordinary. It seems that patients who had the highest degree of resistance to cisplatin—off-the-map levels of resistance—were paradoxically the most sensitive to the combination of cisplatin plus gemcitabine. A true discovery. We came to realize that the very mechanism that these cancer cells used in their defense became an Achilles' heel for their sensitivity to the doublet. Over the years, in collaboration with investigators at the Free University of Amsterdam, we unraveled the mystery of this collateral sensitivity and launched numerous successful clinical trials, all later described in a textbook that we published together (Kroep 2006). But that would be years later and Liz needed my help today.

Despite the three-hour time difference, I decided to call the Pankes at home. It was after 10 PM, Tuesday night, where they lived. Tom answered and Liz got on the phone. "I found the treatment for you," I said.

"Should we come to California for treatment?"

"No." Although the combination was new to this disease, the drugs were widely available. I promised to contact Dr. Ruehlman first thing in the morning (allowing for the time difference) and communicate the schedule I would recommend. They were cautiously optimistic as we ended our conversation.

The next morning, as promised, I came in early and called Dr. Ruehlman in Cincinnati. I introduced myself, explained who I was and what I had done, and asked if he would provide the treatment outlined. He was gracious and thanked me for my interest saying that he would of course utilize the selected drugs, if he could. But the Pankes had already left for California.

Despite my suggestion, their desperation drove them to me for treatment. That afternoon, I met the Pankes for the first time at the Long Beach Memorial Medical Center. Tom was tall, slender, athletic in build and walked with a slight lilt. Liz was desperately ill. She had lost her hair and her eyebrows and her skin had a pale-gray hue. There were dark rings around her eyes. But she looked youthful and very frightened. Nonetheless, she had an air of extraordinary determination and seemed utterly unwilling to yield. Our adventure together was about to begin.

Liz was admitted to the sixth-floor oncology unit. Knowing exactly what I wanted to use, I wrote the orders for the combination of cisplatin plus gemcitabine at the doses and schedules that I had developed years earlier. I then added the same drug combination to be delivered intraperitoneally (placed directly into the abdominal cavity).

Knowing that no one else would consider administering this two-drug combination into the peritoneal cavity, I arrived on the sixth floor and called in a favor by asking Diana Solis from the ultrasound department to assist me in identifying the best spot to insert my drainage catheter needle. Diana, a most dedicated and hardworking ultrasound technician, had become a great ally. Together, we had saved many lives, and when I asked for her assistance, she always complied. With her arrival, I identified a site and aspirated an additional two liters of cancerous fluid. At the same time that I was administering the intravenous dose of cisplatin plus gemcitabine, I used the intraperitoneal needle—still in place from the aspiration—to infuse 30 milligrams of cisplatin and 500 milligrams of gemcitabine directly into the abdominal cavity. Withdrawing the needle and bandaging the wound, I gently kneaded her abdomen and rolled her from side to side to allow the intraperitoneal chemotherapy to reach every surface.

After the intravenous chemotherapy infusion was completed, Liz was hydrated overnight.

The next morning Liz was discharged and she and her husband moved to a hotel nearby. Despite the intensity of the therapy, Liz felt remarkably well. So much so that she and her husband took my recommendation and had dinner downtown at one of my favorite restaurants, La Traviata.

They enjoyed their dinner immensely and, I recall, they bought me a gift certificate in celebration. Within days, Liz was feeling very well. I recommended that this treatment could be administered in Cincinnati and there was no reason for them to continue taking time from their busy schedules to remain in California. After writing the orders, I sent them to her doctor in Cincinnati. I explained that the ascites fluid should begin to ebb. It was my expectation that one additional intraperitoneal cycle would be administered and that access would be provided at the time of paracentesis (the procedure by which fluid is drained from the abdominal cavity through a catheter). I explained to the Pankes that I was hoping and expecting that the fluid would soon thereafter disappear.

Dr. Ruehlman delivered treatment exactly as I prescribed. Each passing day, Liz felt better. On day twenty-two, the beginning of the new cycle of therapy, I received a frantic call. They had arrived at Dr. Ruehlman's office to undergo treatment and the ultrasound technician couldn't find any fluid in the abdomen. Dr. Ruehlman wouldn't be able to deliver the intraperitoneal chemotherapy. It was an odd call. I explained to Tom and Liz that this wasn't bad news. It was good news. No, it was great news. After all, the four liters of fluid that continued to accumulate each week had completely resolved with two weeks of therapy. We had achieved our first goal and now needed only to continue with intravenous treatments. Comforted, she continued with therapy.

Liz achieved a complete remission. All measurable disease and all biochemical parameters returned to normal. Christmas came and went, so did Valentine's Day and Easter. On a routine follow-up with her gynecologist, a small area of abnormality was noted at the suture line of the surgery. A needle aspiration revealed cancer.

We screened Liz high and low with every diagnostic test and could not find evidence of disease anywhere, except in that one small area. Pondering the findings I realized that Liz was suffering from a suture-line recurrence. A scar, from the time of her surgery, had trapped a small number of cells in a fibrous sheath. These cells, shrouded in connective tissue, were impervious to the chemotherapy delivery because, in essence, they had never been exposed.

The option was to re-excise the surgical site or deliver limited radiation. We opted for the radiation with small doses of chemotherapy delivered concurrently to further heighten the radiation effects. By now, Liz was so convinced of my "magical abilities" that she and her husband chose to commute to California to receive the radiation therapy. This well-tolerated combination resulted in the final resolution of all disease.

Liz is now twelve years into complete, durable remission. Fully twelve years after she was told that she would die.

ALIVE TO TELL HER TALE

Not surprisingly, Tom and Liz Panke became champions of our work. But at the time I had no idea how valuable their input would prove to be.

In the fall of 1999, I ran into an old friend, Douglas Blayney, MD, then a member of Wilshire Oncology and some years later the president of the American Society of Clinical Oncology. In our brief discussion at the Phoenix airport, where connecting flights put us momentarily together, he asked whether I was aware of Oncotech's petition to the Department of Health and Human Services (HHS), requesting Medicare approval for its extreme drug resistance

(EDR) assay. Caught completely by surprise, I contacted Dr. Larry Weisenthal and together we approached HHS for information.

We came to learn that Oncotech had crafted a reimbursement schedule that would cover its assay, and its assay only. The fee schedule (at $890 per assay) was inadequate to cover the more sophisticated drug response profiles that we conducted. An approval at this level of reimbursement would have disastrous effects upon our work. On one hand, we would have to accept the Oncotech reimbursement schedule and lose several thousand on every test we conducted. Our other option would be to stop accepting Medicare patients, making it virtually impossible for me, as a clinician, to continue to see patients. After all, my father was a cancer patient; the prospect of being unable to provide him care was distressing indeed. The alternative—e.g. being slowly forced into bankruptcy by Medicare patients—seemed equally unappealing.

How did this all come to pass? Oncotech offered a semi-automated assay method designed to eliminate "inactive" drugs, to which they applied the term "EDR" for Extreme Drug Resistance. Through a series of special analyses and pathology services, they found that they could add enough fees to cover the unprofitable EDR test. For them, it was a lost leader; for us, it was our bread and butter. Our tests were more labor intensive and costly to conduct, with the ability to identify active drugs, not just eliminate inactive ones. While the different assay methods might have distinct applications, we couldn't possibly conduct our business at the fees that Oncotech charged. This was the fight of my life, and I intended to win it.

After conferring with legal counsel, I flew to Baltimore, Maryland, on November 13, 1999, and arrived at the Hyatt to attend the preliminary HHS meeting the next day. For Oncotech, it was the opportunity of a lifetime. If it could obtain an imprimatur of Medicare approval, it could seize the high ground as a federally sanctioned technology, while successfully eliminating the competition by undercutting our reimbursements. It would have been a coup. And, in preparation, Oncotech had paid for investigators from as far away as England to come and promote its work.

When it came to my time to speak, I focused on the distinction between growth-based (Oncotech) and death-based assays, the importance of programmed cell death, and the growing scientific understanding that supported our approach over theirs. Every scientist in the room, of which there were many, congratulated me on a convincing presentation. Yet, the physicians, less familiar with the underlying science, voted in favor of Oncotech. It was a dark day for me and for my chosen field.

I returned to California and sought the opinion of Paul Radenski, MD, JD. Dr. Radenski is a uniquely qualified lawyer whose expertise in regulatory affairs and medical policy is legend. Were my skills in medical oncology to approximate his in medically related legal decision making, I would have long since cured cancer. Dr. Radenski explained the implications of Oncotech's strategy. Were it to succeed it would have the effect of excluding other technologies, leaving Oncotech the heir apparent to cancer chemosensitivity testing.

The stakes were high. The Medicare advisory board meeting in Baltimore, where Oncotech had received approval, could only be implemented if the overlords of Medicare agreed and upheld the recommendation. *That* meeting was to be held in Beltsville, Maryland, outside of Washington.

It was do or die.

I contacted Tom and Liz Panke. By now, a month into treatment, Liz was remarkably well, back at work, and a true believer in our abilities. I asked if they'd allow me to use her case as an example when I attended the meeting in Beltsville. I explained that Oncotech, its CEO, and its scientific advisors would argue for a Medicare coverage decision. Despite my desire to make these tests available to Medicare, I knew that an approval at $890—largely a loss leader for Oncotech who piled on additional service charges to develop fee schedules that were multiples of my charges—would bankrupt me.

I had to win. Medicare would need to reconsider a coverage decision at a level that either increased the fee for all or broke the services down into drug-resistance and drug-sensitivity analyses—the latter reflecting my work.

"Where's the meeting?" Tom asked.

"Beltsville, Maryland," I replied.

"When is it?"

"The day after tomorrow."

"Can I come?" Liz chimed in.

"I don't know. I have been granted an opportunity to speak as a participant and expert, but I don't know who else is allowed to attend."

The committee had provided me copies of Oncotech's reports and I compiled my rebuttal. The next morning the Pankes called and said they'd be there.

"Be where?" I asked.

"Beltsville. I'm an invited speaker," said Liz.

"You're what?"

"I'm an invited speaker. I introduced myself as Elizabeth Panke, MD, PhD, director of the genetic analysis laboratory Genetica, with a personal familiarity in the field, and they granted me five minutes, the same amount of time as everyone else."

I was flabbergasted. I paused for a moment and then inquired, "Didn't you just get your second cycle of chemotherapy?"

"Yes," Liz replied. "Yesterday."

"How can you possibly travel?"

"Easily," she said. "I'm feeling great."

We agreed to meet at a hotel outside of Baltimore on the morning before the session. Bright and early, we had coffee together. Not only did Liz and Tom pay their own airfare and hotel, but they would not allow me to buy them breakfast, fearing even the slightest perception of impropriety. We traveled together by cab, from the hotel to the Beltsville facility, dividing the fare down the middle.

Entering the hall, we saw there were speakers from the Brookings Institute, universities, biotech labs, as well as dozens of other experts, all seated on a large, semicircular stage. The amphitheater was filled with interested parties: insurers, scientists, doctors. On the schedule were a number of different medical services seeking Medicare coverage.

Very sophisticated discussions of medical data, outcomes, quality of life, costs reimbursement, and performance characteristics ensued. Preceding our presentation (the last of the day) was a consortium of bone marrow transplant experts who were seeking Medicare coverage for their procedure for treatment of multiple myeloma. The data seemed compelling—that is, until one of the experts on the stage pointed out that not a single patient in any of the studies reported had been over sixty-five years of age. As only patients sixty-five years of age and older are covered by Medicare, the studies were deemed inadmissible and approval was denied.

Now it was our turn. Frank Kiesner, CEO of Oncotech, David Kern, laboratory director, and John Freuhauf, medical director, all spoke, as did my colleague and collaborator Larry Weisenthal (who was engaged in studies similar to my own). Oddly, and for reasons that to this day I am not sure I understand, Dr. Weisenthal argued in favor of Oncotech's approval. I found myself the only voice opposing the approval process. I gave my presentation and remember distinctly describing their approval of this single technology for coverage being tantamount to "forcing the entire field of drug sensitivity testing onto a procrustean bed." The reference was to "Procrustes," the figure in Greek mythology who strapped unwary guests to his bed. If they were too tall, he cut off their legs. If they were too short, he stretched them to size. The term is used to describe overly restrictive covenants. My allegorical reference appeared to resonate with one of the reviewers on the stage who nodded to me approvingly. My five minutes were up—I had made my appeal.

The conference organizer then called Dr. Elizabeth Panke of

Genetica to the microphone. Across the gallery, where the interested parties were seated, I heard a resounding, "Who?"

Liz, neatly coiffed in a wig and a smart business suit, walked to the microphone. She explained that she was a molecular biologist, that she had been diagnosed with an untreatable malignancy and, a month earlier, had been given a death sentence. Learning belatedly of the field of drug sensitivity testing, she explained that she'd submitted a tissue sample both to Oncotech and to my laboratory. She went on to say that the Oncotech assay, designed to identify drug resistance, whatever its merits or deficiencies, had provided her with an utterly useless recommendation. The EDR (extreme drug resistance) analysis recommended that she should receive the exact same three drugs that had just failed her. She then described that the more discriminating cell-death-based assay applied by our laboratory had recommended a novel two-drug combination, which had provided her the first meaningful benefit and clinical response since her original diagnosis five months earlier. She was there today, standing before them, not because a drug resistance assay had helped her, but because a drug sensitivity assay had identified a life-saving therapy. She concluded that a broad-brush approval, that restricted reimbursement through Medicare to the "lowest common denominator" assay technology, would stifle progress and lead to the deaths of countless patients just like her. Denied the advantages of truly discriminating endpoints, these patients would confront the same grim outcome she so narrowly avoided. She thanked the experts and sat down.

Several people in the audience stood up and shook her hand. The reviewers were visibly moved. It was late. The committee members were polled. They agreed that the preliminary committee's findings from the previous month had been incomplete; that the field was manifestly more complex; and that a Medicare approval decision at this time would be premature. Oncotech's application for Medicare approval was denied.

Liz Panke had carried the day.

16

Progress in Treating Kidney Cancer

In the field of medical oncology some forms of cancer are bad, others are worse, and then there's kidney cancer (also known as renal cell carcinoma). Because the kidney is an organ that is designed to filter the blood of impurities, it is armed with a number of defenses that enable it to process and excrete these toxins.

Among these defenses are an abundance of efflux pumps—energy-driven, one-way valves (proteins), which actively pass chemicals from the inside of the cell to the outside. It so happens that these proteins are closely related to drug-resistance mechanisms associated with the overexpression of one specific protein, p-glycoprotein. Decades of research have focused upon p-glycoprotein and related phenomena as the cause of chemotherapy resistance in cancer.

In addition, kidney cells are rich in the sulfur-containing amino acid cysteine. Cysteine makes up the business end of one of the most important detoxifying substances in cells known as glutathione. These and other features of kidney cells make them almost impervious to the effects of chemotherapy following malignant transformation. As a result, renal cell carcinoma has remained one of the most challenging forms of cancer that medical oncologists confront.

Until a few years ago, there was virtually nothing available for these patients. Metastatic disease was associated with virtually no response to therapy. While the literature included occasional successes with progesterone, vinblastine, and time-sequenced administration of 5-FU (chronomodulated), for the most part once someone was diagnosed with advanced kidney cancer his or her outcome was written in stone. And then along came the discovery that these highly vascular kidney cancers, arising in an organ that is itself responsible for the regulation of red blood cell growth (through a protein known as erythropoietin), could be attacked by antivascular therapies. The first successful therapy for renal carcinoma was the monoclonal antibody bevacizumab, known commercially as Avastin, which blocks the vascular growth factor VEGF. Then came sunitinib and sorafenib. These oral medications worked inside the cell to short-circuit the same signal that Avastin targeted.

After decades of no success, by 2005 there were three active drugs in the market for the treatment of kidney cancer. Today, newly diagnosed patients are offered the drug sunitinib. Sold under the commercial name Sutent, this relatively well-tolerated oral therapy is the gold standard for metastatic renal cell carcinoma today. Virtually all patients receive it as their first-line therapy.

But what happens when sunitinib fails to work? For some patients, a second-line therapy with the closely related sorafenib provides benefit, while other patients, smaller in number, may respond to the newer classes of drugs known as mTOR inhibitors. None of these second-line therapies are highly effective and the majority of patients fail to show any objective response.

In September 2010, John Friedberg, MD, an accomplished neurologist and published author from Berkeley, California, found himself confronting metastatic renal cell carcinoma that had spread from his right kidney to both of his lungs and, worst of all, was rapidly progressing despite sunitinib therapy. However exciting the new frontier of therapeutics in kidney cancer might be, Dr. Friedberg was going down in flames.

While working in my laboratory one afternoon, my assistant came in to ask if I'd take a call from a physician who was calling from Stanford. I got up from my microscope and walked to the phone, where

I encountered a craggy-voiced gentleman who was obviously short of breath. He introduced himself and explained that he was in the radiology department at Stanford Medical Center, where an interventional radiologist was about to draw fluid from his lung. Having come across reference to my work, Dr. Friedberg inquired whether we could process the pleural fluid about to be removed from his lung. "Of course," I said. He handed the phone to the radiologist, and I explained the procedure of processing the fluid.

The next day, the fluid arrived at my laboratory. But, alas, there were no cancer cells to be found when we processed the material. When we contacted Dr. Friedberg to explain our findings, he said, "I'm coming down there for a biopsy." He hung up.

Two days later, a dark silver Prius pulled into the Rational Therapeutics' parking lot. Out stepped a young woman wearing long black-and-white striped socks. *Pippi Longstocking,* I remember thinking to myself. She moved around to the other side of the car and assisted Dr. Friedberg into our waiting room. He was shown to my office and sat down, quite breathless.

There was an air of desperation and fear in his voice. But he was absolutely determined to have me conduct an assay on his tissue. After examining him, recognizing that both lungs were filled with fluid, I noted a large lymph node in the right armpit. He pointed to it and said that he wanted the lump removed and for us to study it on his behalf. I pride myself on offering even the most ill patients the opportunity to get better. I sometimes tread where others fear to go. But, in this case, I was afraid to biopsy the patient. He was so ill, so debilitated, so pale, so gaunt, so short of breath. I couldn't imagine he could get through a biopsy, much less tolerate any treatment, whatever I might find.

I explained my misgivings, but Dr. Friedberg would hear none of it. He looked me in the eye and said, "I am a doctor and I know better than most what it means if you can't help me. You need to do this biopsy."

I was conflicted. I want to help everyone. But this was a tough call. I did everything I could to explain the risks and hazards, the unlikelihood of a good outcome, the toxicities of the treatments we might find, and all the rest. It did no good. He was going for a biopsy and that was that. We arranged for a colleague to conduct the axillary biopsy. The patient came through it without difficulty, and he and Pippi Longstocking climbed back into the Prius and returned home.

I remember hoping I had done the right thing.

I later came to realize that Dr. Friedberg was almost immediately hospitalized upon his return to Berkeley. It seems that in addition to the hardships his cancer wrought, he was also suffering from a tumor-related autoimmune hemolytic anemia that was chewing through his red cells faster than he could make them.

His medical oncologist, Gary Cecchi, MD, contacted me. I remember the conversation well. He explained that he had known Dr. Friedberg for years, that he was newly aware of his management through Stanford and appreciated my efforts on his colleague's behalf. Dr. Cecchi had a slightly gruff quality, a tough guy sound, like someone from New Jersey, which is where he turned out to be from. With my analysis in hand, I explained to Dr. Cecchi the combination we had identified for Dr. Friedberg.

"You want me to give him what?" said Cecchi.

"Low-dose cisplatin plus gemcitabine with oral xeloda."

"You don't understand," he responded. "This guy is dying."

"I understand very well," I told him. "I just saw him a couple of days ago and I agree, but this is what he wants and I don't have the heart to say no. I'd appreciate it if you'd work with me here."

Luckily, Dr. Cecchi agreed and started the recommended treatment. To say things got rocky would be a gross understatement. Dr. Friedberg wound up in the ICU with a hemoglobin count that rarely got north of seven (normal is 13–14), severe fluid retention, and an inability to get enough oxygen. He required massive transfusions and lapsed in and out of a state of confused delirium.

About two weeks later, I received a phone call. It was Dr. Friedberg. His voice was stronger. He had been transferred from the ICU to a medical ward. His transfusion requirements had diminished. He was breathing better. And, amazingly, his x-ray was better. A few weeks later, Dr. Friedberg was home, off oxygen, enjoying the visits from his Yorkshire terrier, Buddy, and receiving his second cycle of the chemotherapy regimen I had outlined for him. By now, he was very much better: eating, gaining weight, and beginning to carry on normal activities. From early October through mid-November 2010, he had made a dramatic rebound.

A short time after that, his CT scan was repeated. What I describe now doesn't happen very often. I got a call from Dr. Cecchi. He was beside himself. He went on and on saying, "I've never seen anything like it. I've never seen a solid tumor melt away like this. I mean, maybe in lymphoma, but never, ever kidney cancer."

Dr. Friedberg was dramatically better. We encouraged him to continue his treatments. And then, in late January 2011, we received an email. It was a photograph taken at Donner Ski Ranch, the resort located in Lake Tahoe, California. A slight man, dressed in a snowboard jacket, was holding a small dog in his arm. Upon closer inspection, I realized that it was Dr. Friedberg. He was snowboarding!

With each successive course of therapy, Dr. Friedberg's tumor shrank until there was nothing left other than the mass in the right kidney. Dr. Friedberg wanted the kidney removed. This was uncharted territory. It was one thing to change the course of mighty rivers and bend steel with your bare hands, but it was quite another to travel at the speed of light. Dr. Friedberg was asking the impossible. Could we even possibly, remotely contemplate curing this patient? Could we remove the tumor that remained in his kidney and in so doing render him free of disease?

Dr. Friedberg was insistent. He wanted it out. He went so far as to obtain opinions from several surgeons. He had become an unstoppable force. By this time it was no longer a discussion of whether to have surgery, but instead, whether it was going to be open or laparoscopic. On April 18, 2011, the surgery was conducted and the remaining tumor was submitted to our laboratory. Interestingly, the residual disease retained a profile of drug sensitivity that was virtually identical to the original biopsy. We encouraged Dr. Friedberg to continue postoperative treatment; he complied and continued receiving maintenance therapy.

He regained his normal weight, fully healed from surgery, and returned to his normal activities. The best news of all was the normal PET scan Dr. Friedberg obtained in July 2011.

In celebration of our patients and to support the needs of medically indigent patients, the Vanguard Cancer Foundation holds an annual fundraiser in Los Angeles. Our 2011 event was held on October 1 at a famous old chophouse in the City of Commerce—Stevens Steak and Seafood House. Dr. Friedberg kindly offered to attend and I, in return, asked if he would speak. Standing before the assembled crowd of more than 300 guests, Dr. Friedberg described the depth of his illness and the miracle of his good outcome. He was funny, charming, and iconoclastic. He spoke of his experiences at Stanford and of his physicians there—who apparently lost interest in his good outcome. He spoke of his utter dismay that our laboratory work is not more widely used. He said how glad he was to be there that night . . . not just there at Stevens Steak and Seafood House, but alive, there on the planet. In his parting shot, he quoted the famous exercise and nutrition guru Jack LaLanne, who, when asked about his own mortality replied, "I can't afford to die, it'll wreck my image."

Just as Jack LaLanne, the father of modern health consciousness, could not live forever, dying at the age of ninety-six on January 24, 2011, John Friedberg too lost his battle with cancer at the second year. In the end, it wasn't our failure or that of his physicians, but instead a lack of active drugs, both cytotoxic and targeted, that sealed his fate. Despite our best efforts, a repeat biopsy yielded no leads. Our quiver was empty. There were no arrows left.

17

Ah, the Simple Life

The 1960s Scottish musical group Incredible String Band had a tune about the life of an amoeba called "A Very Cellular Song." The final verse reads:

> *If I need a friend I just give a wriggle,*
> *Split right down the middle.*
> *And when I look there's two of me,*
> *Both as handsome as can be.*

This whimsical depiction of primordial existence reflects the life of single cell organisms. They don't have lungs or livers, blood supplies or brains. There are no arms and legs, no hands and feet, no eyes, no ears. There's just one cell.

At this level, life constitutes a continuous and inescapable interaction with the environment. The amoeba's life is little more than consumption, elimination, and replication. The amoeba tracks its food sources and slithers to the dinner table. Once full, it splits down the middle and where there was one, there are two. Such was life for more than a billion years. And then, organisms got together.

First, they do so through a process known as endosymbiosis, originally described by Lynn Margulis who theorized that mitochondria—found in every cell—were nothing more than bacteria that hitched a ride within the cell. The mitochondria offer up energy (as ATP) to the cell in return for mobility, protection, and a steady source of nutrients.

This symbiosis at the cellular level was then replicated at the multicellular level. Single cells joined together and specialized. The outer layer provided protection; the inner layer provided reproductive capacity and metabolic activity. As organisms became more complex, the specialization grew.

Once organisms achieved a given size, simple diffusion (passive movement) could no longer provide the foodstuffs and oxygen needed by the inner layers. Blood supplies were developed to transport nutrients, and lungs came into existence to oxygenate the blood. Finally, a nervous system was required to coordinate and integrate functions.

Despite the increasing complexity of these interacting networks, individual cells continued to rely upon many of the same metabolic processes that sustain the amoeba. Glycolysis (the basic metabolism of sugars) and oxidative phosphorylation (secondary metabolism that takes place within the mitochondria, also known as the Krebs cycle) are virtually the same in every living cell. How, then, do multicellular organisms maintain control over the masses of cells now numbering in the trillions?

Each cell remembers its origins only too well. It wants mobility, a food supply, and protection. The dilemma of the metazoan (multicellular organism) is to control the unlimited wants of these seething mobs.

The organism as a whole offers each cell protection and nutrients, extracting in return a promise of absolute obedience. Every cell is given a job and those jobs must be fulfilled in their entirety—not more or less than asked.

To govern these selfish cells, the body uses growth factors. These are like small morsels of nectar doled out judiciously to the individual cells at the behest of the organism as a whole. Any cell that fails to do its job sees its nutrients withdrawn and its life terminated. These growth factors come in many varieties—epidermal growth factor, insulin-like growth factor, hepatocyte growth factor, and vascular endothelial growth factor. In other words, "Play ball by my rules, or you don't play at all."

But cancer breaks the contract. Cancer wants to stay out all night and steal your lunch. If it sticks to the rules, its privileges are curtailed and its ultimate success is limited. To escape these constraints, cancers break the shackles of growth factors. Activating mutations in signaling proteins known as kinases, or expanding the pools of available growth factors themselves, allows cancers to escape control. They no longer play by the rules. They can pull sugar and proteins directly out of the blood supply even if martial law has been declared. Cancer is on a bender and it's party time.

This new understanding has come under the term "metabolomics." The cancer research community left the fields of metabolism, biochemistry, and enzymology during the 1950s to pursue the developing field of genomics. It is ironic, however, that the discoveries of genomics have now dragged the molecular biologists back to metabolism, biochemistry, and enzymology.

If one attends the most sophisticated scientific conferences today, the hot topics being covered are pyruvate kinase, alpha-ketoglutarate, fumarate hydratase and the process of glutaminolysis. These molecules, enzymes, and pathways, uncovered through modern genomic analyses, are nothing more than the machinery of metabolism. Not a single presentation goes by without the investigators referencing that very modern and groundbreaking paper written by Otto Warburg, originally published in 1930. It was in this paper that Warburg described "aerobic glycolysis," the process by which cancers forgo energetically advantageous mitochondrial metabolism in favor of the comparatively less efficient glucose consumption in the cytoplasm. Unraveling the reasons why will be the subject of years of future research.

THE FUTURE OF CANCER RESEARCH LIES BEHIND US

What our forays into the gene have taught us is that the genetic abnormalities of cancer, those causative events, are, in fact, really changes in cellular metabolism. Further, these changes offer opportunities for therapy. Therapies that interrupt or block signaling pathways that communicate from the outside world (the cell membrane) to the inside world (the nucleus) are now known as targeted therapies.

Earlier forms of cancer therapy, designed to interrupt nuclear function and mitosis (cell division) targeted DNA for damage. Yet, the Achilles' heel of cancer is not the reproductive capacities found in the DNA, but instead the very same processes that lead amoebas to seek out sugar. Cancer cells are looking for nothing more than three hots and a cot, and it turns out that our most advanced therapies today are little more than diet plans.

Indeed, one of the most important pathways in cancer is the insulin-like growth factor pathway. Insulin, that sugar-regulating protein, and its close counterpart, insulin-like growth factor, are among the most important survival signals in biology. A cell given insulin will grow, absorb nutrients, alter its metabolism, and outlive its neighbors.

Disrupting this pathway at the level of the cell membrane receptor or at several points downstream has become the battle cry of oncologic therapeutics. As we peel back the layers of complexity associated with cancer-causing syndromes, we find them to be little more than perturbations in cellular metabolism and survival benefits.

Thus, our investment in genomics, $3 billion and counting, has brought us squarely back to where we were in the 1930s, 1940s, and 1950s before we discovered the double helix structure of DNA. Imagine what other future discoveries lay behind us.

18

What to Do When
Your Genes Don't Fit

I t had long been a puzzle why young women developed aggressive breast and ovarian cancers. No one knew why these cancers
occurred in families and why many of those families were of East-
ern European, Jewish heritage. In 1992, Mary Claire King, PhD,
solved that puzzle when she described the BRCA1 and BRCA2
gene mutations, named for the breast cancer predisposition with
which they were associated. Screening programs were soon developed and today we are very aware of the risks associated with these
mutations.

But what of the patients whose diagnoses came long before the
description of these genes? One such patient was Sharon Williamson. Her saga began in 1971, with her first diagnosis of breast cancer. She underwent surgery and chemotherapy. By the late 1970s,
she had her second breast cancer and was again treated with surgery and chemotherapy. Years later, she developed ovarian cancer.
Again, surgery and chemotherapeutics were able to render her
disease-free.

A subsequent recurrence of her ovarian cancer in the mid 1990s
was again managed with chemotherapy with good response. It was
with this occurrence that her physician submitted Sharon for a
BRCA analysis. Her results revealed a heretofore unrecognized
BRCA1 deletion mutation (a portion of DNA removed from the

gene) that proved responsible for her cancer predisposition. Sharon and her family members, who carried the same deletion mutation, became the subjects of a published manuscript that described this unusual finding (Gad 2001).

In retrospect, it should have been obvious that Sharon carried a mutation. After all, she had her first diagnosis of breast cancer at age thirty and ovarian cancer at age forty-nine. More to the point, one sister was diagnosed with breast cancer at the age of thirty-five, while her second sister was diagnosed with ovarian cancer, also at thirty-five. Sharon was a cancer time bomb.

By the time I met her in 2002, she had already undergone bilateral mastectomies, a hysterectomy, and multiple courses of chemotherapy. She requested our input regarding her most recent recurrence of ovarian cancer. A biopsy was obtained and revealed activity for a combination of cisplatin plus gemcitabine. This combination was the subject of prior studies by our group and was gaining attention in the literature. Her response was prompt and dramatic, but her tolerance rapidly dwindled.

During the first year of treatment, her blood counts failed to recover and doses needed adjustment. Then we began to widen out the schedules two weeks, three weeks, four weeks. Despite these adjustments, we were rapidly exhausting her bone marrow reserves.

Concerned by the cytotoxic drug side effects, I returned to my original analyses of Sharon's tumor. In addition to the cisplatin plus gemcitabine doublet, she had an excellent profile for a combination that I had never given to a patient with ovarian cancer: vinorelbine plus capecitabine. The regimen, previously described for treatment of breast cancer, had not been used in gynecologic malignancies. Yet, we had ongoing research that supported meaningful synergy and efficacy for this combination in ovarian cancer patients (Brewer 2008).

With our options limited, it was worth a shot. My colleagues in gynecologic oncology, who had kindly supported Sharon through her cisplatin plus gemcitabine treatments, had never heard of nor had ever given my new combination, and were not comfortable administering it. We were on our own.

Sharon transferred her care to me and I initiated therapy. I remember how frail she seemed. Her blood counts were low, resulting in wound infections of the chest wall. The platinum-based chemotherapy had taken its toll. The new treatment was started, and she perked up immediately. At low doses, the vinorelbine had almost no toxicity and the capecitabine, taken by mouth, was a cinch. Within a few cycles, her CA125 had normalized. So did her initial PET scan and every subsequent PET scan. Year after year after year, Sharon's CA125, PET scan, and all other indicators of disease remained within normal limits.

My colleague in nuclear medicine began to complain that Sharon's repeat studies were becoming boring. He would deflect my repeated efforts to explain the miraculous nature of this durable remission. "Yeah, yeah, I know. The lady who failed everything who is still in remission five years later," Jeff Dobkin, MD, would jokingly say.

Interestingly, it was the same gene mutation that caused Sharon to develop cancer that proved her salvation. The BRCA1 and 2 mutations are known as "genomic fidelity genes." Their role is to recognize and repair DNA damage. Under normal conditions, these genes cobble together the necessary response elements to clear the DNA of dangerous abnormalities and return the genes to their normal state. The absence of these genes (mutation), as was the case in Sharon, renders normal tissues at risk for unrepaired mutations. Over a life of wear and tear, the accumulation of abnormalities results in cancer. The good news is that these cancers carry with them the same inability to repair DNA damage. This renders them hypersensitive to certain types of therapy—like radiation, platinum, and alkylator-based treatments, as well as the DNA look-alikes like 5-FU and gemcitabine, known as antimetabolites.

We had stumbled upon the Achilles' heel of Sharon's tumor and used it to good effect. What was so gratifying about her case was that the toxicity seemed almost exclusively suffered by the tumor. Sharon never felt sick, lost her hair, or stopped living an absolutely normal life. From vacations in Hawaii to tours of the Galapagos Islands, she and her husband, Dale, never missed a beat.

Sadly, fate would have it that the many years of radiation and mutation-inducing chemotherapies finally caught up with Sharon. Her ovarian cancer never recurred. Nor did her breast cancers. Instead, she developed a smoldering form of leukemia known as myelodysplasia. When we examined the bone marrow, she had so many accumulated mutations that virtually no normal marrow function remained. Within weeks of the initial diagnosis she was hospitalized, and days later, she died.

If there were ever a Pyrrhic victory in medicine (from Pyrrhus, whose victory over the Romans in the battle of Asculum in 279 BC so decimated his troops that he could not continue to wage war—win-lose scenario), Sharon was the poster child. The very treatments that she had received to prolong her life, from 1971 onward, had sealed her fate. I cannot for a moment fault the physicians who treated her for her original diagnoses. Each decade that those therapies prolonged her life was a victory. Yet, Sharon's ultimate demise from myelodysplasia, the result of these treatments, reminds us that cytotoxic chemotherapy is a double-edged sword with a razor-sharp back edge.

WHAT GENOMICS IS AND WHAT IT ISN'T

On April 25, 1953, a brief paper appeared in the journal *Nature* (Watson 1953) that described the double helix structure of DNA. With this discovery, the mystery of genetic information became demonstrably clearer.

What Watson and Crick had shown was that the DNA bases (the building blocks of DNA) aligned themselves in a highly specific manner—guanine to cytosine and adenine to thymine—along a railroad track of information. The DNA and RNA polymerases (enzymes that read the DNA code) transcribe the information and prepare the cell for action. With each passing year, new discoveries brought us ever closer to the brink of a complete understanding of human biology. Or so we thought.

Human biology is many things, but simple isn't one of them. We are, as a species, indeed as living things, much more than the sum of our genes. The information contained in the gene does not determine what you will be, but instead is permissive. Without a gene you cannot express the feature. But having a gene does not dictate that you *will* express the feature.

In 2003, the culmination of the genomic revolution was upon us—the sequencing of the entire human genome. But even this great revolution has not cured cancer. We know the address and the next-door neighbors of every human gene, yet we don't know what they do, how they do it, why they do it, or who they do it with. Simply put, the human genome project has provided us the world's most expensive telephone book.

Human discovery plays out similarly in many disciplines. We are witness to a not dissimilar experience in space exploration. It took centuries for us to develop the first airplane; within decades we had jets and a decade later we had rockets capable of achieving orbit around the earth. The slow, steady development of our understanding of heavier-than-air travel and productive application of Bernoulli's principle (the faster a gas or liquid moves, the lower the pressure) might have, under other circumstances, led us to develop a space-going jet plane. But around the same time that we discovered the structure of DNA, the Soviet Union sent *Sputnik* into space and all bets were off.

"I, for one, do not want to sleep by the light of a Communist moon," said then Senator Lyndon B. Johnson in October 1957, decrying the Soviets' lead in space exploration.

The race was on. We were going to get to space one way or another and the smooth trajectory that led from airplane to jet to super orbital jet was suddenly hijacked by devotees of the slingshot.

Instead of working to develop a supersonic jet aircraft that could fly into space and return under the control of a pilot, we catapulted first one, then two, and finally three astronauts at a time into the atmosphere atop Saturn rockets. Their brief forays into space ended with them falling back, under Earth's gravitational pull, only to be rescued, bobbing helplessly in the ocean.

Decade after decade we launched our brave astronauts into space with no lasting impact and no meaningful advances in the technology that would make true space exploration a success. Recognizing the shortcomings of this approach, NASA rededicated itself to a manned space vehicle and in 1981 launched the first space shuttle.

So what's this got to do with cancer? Quite a lot, it seems.

Cancer research over centuries had focused upon the chemistry of life. The mysteries of cancer were slowly being explored through the dedicated efforts of biochemists and enzymologists (scientists who study proteins known as enzymes, which are responsible for most biochemical reactions). Their hard-fought discoveries led to our understanding of oxidative phosphorylation (the energy production process), membrane physiology (lipid protein interaction), and ionic fluxes (positive and negative ion transfer), as vehicles of cellular communication. These pioneering scientists were moving along the course of discovery that might well have led to much greater understanding today had we not been dazzled by the discovery of DNA's double helix. As we peered behind the kimono of human genomics, hoping to catch a glimpse of the secrets held therein, we unwittingly abdicated the process of scientific discovery to the quick-and-dirty artists known as molecular biologists.

Their modus operandi reflected little more than sophisticated pattern recognition—beginning with the process of DNA gel electrophoresis (which separates DNA components into discrete patterns) all the way to contemporary heat maps of gene expression (color-coded diagrams that define levels of gene expression through a process known as hierarchical clustering). Today, we can run an Oncotype DX or MammaPrint and tell by the pattern obtained the relative likelihood of a good or bad outcome for a breast cancer patient. Yet, we have no idea why these particular patterns confer specific prognoses. Molecular genomics provides a veneer of information that has seduced our best scientists into the false belief that they know more than they really do.

In parallel with our NASA colleagues, we jumped off the biochemistry track (as they did off the manned-aircraft track) and dove headlong into the gene. Today, we realize what an error this may have been. Over the past several years, genomics publications are slowly being replaced by metabolomics publications. Metabolomics is the study of human metabolism at the level of enzyme and biochemical reaction. Scientists are slowly becoming scientists again. Recognizing the shortcomings of information for information's sake, the molecular biologists, who thought they could leave their chemistry books behind and never open them again, are scrambling to relearn the basics.

It turns out that cancer isn't—in the truest sense of the word—a genetic disease. It is, instead, a metabolic disorder. Cancer cells, like all members of multicellular organisms, function under the controlling influence of the organism as a whole. The social contract of cellular biology dictates that each individual cell in a multicellular organism relinquishes its autonomy in return for the provision of nutrients, water, oxygen, protection, and mobility. But cancer cells break the contract and escape the regulatory control so essential for orderly multicellular existence.

Viewing cancer in this light, where we once saw cells as proteins and lipids driven by the information contained in their DNA, and defined them by their capacity for self-replication, we must now view these microscopic entities as complex biosystems that retrieve information from their DNA the way computers draw upon their disk drives. While computer scientists would bristle at the idea that their field was little more than a floppy disc, modern cancer researchers have succeeded in convincing the public that life equals DNA.

It was our ill-conceived love affair with genomics that led us to the failed war on cancer, and it will be our renewed appreciation of biochemistry that digs us out of this mess. Like the *Apollo 13* astronauts who realized late in the game that they needed to be pilots, scientists today are realizing that they must return to the fundamental principles of physiology, chemistry, and biology to unravel the mysteries of cancer.

LOTS OF HEAT, NO LIGHT

Among the most widely used platforms for the analysis of genetic phenomena are silicon chips that provide what are known as heat maps. These graphic depictions use color codes to break down genetic expressions into over- and underexpressed elements. These heat map graphic depictions provide color-coded gene expression data: red for over- and green for underexpressed. In their own way, they're kind of pretty, like a molecular Rothko painting. For me, the term "heat map" is ironic, as a common usage in heady discussions is the catchphrase "lots of heat, no light."

When I consider genomic analysis, the term that comes to mind is "solipsist." Solipsism is the philosophical school that teaches that the self is the only thing that can be verified, the only reality. The simplest example is the child who believes the world goes away when he closes his eyes. To the molecular geneticist, the truth can only be found in silicon—the platform utilized in gene studies that uses silicon-based chips to provide electric signals when genes of interest are identified. To these investigators, the guiding principle is, "if you can't probe it on a gene chip, it isn't worth knowing about."

Where these intrepid investigators have gone wrong is their failure to recognize that biology is not linear. There is no direct relationship between genes and behavior. When two parents have children and one of the parents has blue eyes, all of the offspring may have brown eyes. We have recognized this since the time of

Gregor Mendel (the father of modern genetics known as Mendelian genetics) as dominant and recessive traits. What we now realize is that gene expression is under immensely complex control. As such, the brown-eyed child may carry a blue-eyed gene. Yet, her eyes are unequivocally brown. Were a molecular biologist to study that child's genetic makeup, they would find a blue-eyed gene. And, judging from current tendencies, they would spend the rest of eternity attempting to convince the child that her brown eyes were blue. Crystal Gayle's 1977 hit ("Don't It Make My Brown Eyes Blue") not withstanding, the "genes don't lie" dictum would soon grow tiresome.

While genes may not lie, their messengers often do. Or they get lost on the way and never express the feature defined by the sequence of DNA. "Central dogma" was the term applied to the concept that genetic information was a one-way street; namely, that DNA made RNA and RNA made protein. What has stymied this otherwise tidy collection of principles are the complexities now recognized as epigenetics.

As stated earlier, genetic findings are not predictive, they are permissive. If you don't carry a gene, you can't express the feature. But the fact that you carry the gene by no means dictates that you will express the feature. That realization is making the people who spent $3 billion on the human genome project a bit uncomfortable. Let's examine for a moment how you become you.

Organisms known as deuterostomes—including the vertebrates, like humans—undergo a carefully scripted program of cell development. Beginning with the fertilized ovum (zygote), each successive series of cell divisions adds an additional layer throughout embryonic development—from morula to blastula and finally gastrula, the earliest stages of multi-cellular growth. By the eighth week of gestation, the organism is recognized as a fetus. With each division, the cells pass on their full complement of genetic material in the form of their DNA code. Everything that can ever be is written in that code. After a series of cell divisions, however, the pluripotent cells (capable of differentiating into any cellular type), now frequently referred to as stem cells, begin the process of genetic restriction, thereby limiting their capabilities to a select few features. Over time, one collection of cells starts expressing the skin pigment melanin and stops expressing the gene for the oxygen-carrying molecule hemoglobin. Another collection of cells starts making hydrochloric acid but no longer retains the capacity to produce tears. These events are regulated through a process known as epigenetics.

Epigenetics, as a field of science, began in the 1950s and 1960s when a series of observations at Cold Spring Harbor and Harvard University established, beyond a shadow of a doubt, that there were heritable features in biology that were not directly coded in the DNA. It became evident to these pioneering investigators that we had the capacity to regulate genetic expression without leaving written clues. The addition of methyl groups (single-carbon fragments) to cytosine bases in DNA, coats the underlying genes with a residue that prevents their expression. At the same time, enzymes add or remove acetate molecules (the acid form of which makes up vinegar) from the proteins that wrap around DNA (the histones). These processes in aggregate turn genes on and off, creating the final product. In essence, the genes are there for the taking, but the body carefully regulates who gets to play. By layering methyl or acetate groups onto the genes, using nuclear enzymes, the cell controls which gene products will ever see the light of day.

Within decades of these discoveries, scientists were examining measurements of epigenetics and developing small molecules that could influence these processes. Drugs like azacytidine and SAHA, inhibitors of these epigenetic processes, are now in clinical practice for the treatment of select malignancies, like myelodysplastic syndrome, a form of preleukemia and cutaneous lymphoma, a cancer that arises in the skin.

With this new and somewhat humbling recognition that it wasn't "all in the genes," the molecular biologists picked themselves up and started anew. "It was *almost* all in the genes," and there was just this tiny little wrinkle called epigenetics. They all had that pretty well under control. At least so they thought, until 1998.

For it was in 1998 that we discovered small interfering RNAs (ribonucleic acids).

What are small interfering RNAs and what do they do? Quite a lot, it turns out.

As you may recall, central dogma dictated that DNA made RNA and RNA made protein. The role of the RNA was to carry the message from DNA to protein. The name given to these couriers was messenger RNA (or mRNA). What we hadn't realized before 1998 was that the path from DNA to protein was fraught with hazards. These hazards, in the form of small interfering RNAs (siRNA), function like linebackers tackling the messenger RNAs as they head for the goal line (in this case, the cell's cytoplasm and the production of an active protein). Just like the game of football, when the mRNA is tackled by an siRNA, the play ends with no goal and everyone returns to the huddle. The process begins anew with the hope that the next play will outmaneuver the tackles and will result in the production of a functional protein.

So, after the DNA has been expressed and all the epigenetic hurdles overcome, and the mRNA is on the launch pad, along come small interfering RNAs and shut the whole process down like a lightning storm over Cape Canaveral just as the shuttle is preparing for launch. And it turns out that this happens often. Very often.

Indeed, 20 percent of all human gene expression is under direct control of small interfering RNAs; another 30 percent is under partial control. This means 50 percent of all of human gene expression is under the regulation of a process that we didn't know anything about before 1998.

Now that we know about epigenetics, DNA methylation, histone acetylation, and small interfering RNAs, can't we just go back to our Affymetrics silicon chips and study genes again? Well, not so fast.

In June 2010, a paper appeared in the journal *Nature* (Poliseno 2010) that undermined even the most devout adherents to molecular genetics belief systems. The report by Pier Paolo Pandolfi, MD, examined the role of noncoding DNA in human biology. Some have heard the term "junk DNA" used to describe the 98 percent of human genetic material that doesn't appear to code for functional proteins. What Dr. Pandolfi found was that at least half of this genetic material was, in fact, being transcribed into messenger RNA. But why would a system as elegant and efficient as the human cell seemingly spin its wheels producing messenger RNAs that never produce proteins?

Pandolfi confirmed that messenger RNAs bind to small interfering RNAs as had been described before. He showed that each time a messenger RNA bound to a small interfering RNA, both the mRNA and the small interfering RNA were removed from the nucleus. Up to that point, Pandolfi's findings were not particularly noteworthy. Where it got interesting was Pandolfi's examination of those DNA sequences that didn't ultimately produce proteins. These are known as "noncoding DNA" for their lack of functional products. It so happens that these noncoding DNA sequences, known as pseudogenes, produce messenger RNAs just like their coding counterparts. These mRNAs peel off the chromosome and run smack-dab into the small interfering RNAs orbiting the genes. Just like their coding brethren, they combine with the small interfering RNAs and are removed from the nucleus. Thus, the noncoding mRNAs compete for the small interfering RNAs and, when enough small interfering RNAs are taken out of commission, the functional mRNAs skip past the linebackers and escape to the cytoplasm where their protein products are produced.

I was dumbfounded. The thought that noncoding DNA sequences produced mRNAs that regulated other mRNAs left me grasping for a handle on reality.

Reading this article had the same effect upon me that my first understanding of the process of apoptosis had had many years earlier. It was a shot across the bow of everything I had come to know and understand of molecular biology. In an instant, the role of DNA had been eclipsed. Suddenly, life had become a function of RNA regulating RNA. Central dogma went out the window and nuclear informatics (information science) had suddenly grown demonstrably more complex. And we hadn't even left the nucleus.

Among the most vexing issues that molecular biologists now confront is the realization that life is not simply a function of informatics. All of the DNA, RNA, small interfering RNAs, and associated pseudogenes are the beginning, not the end, of cellular characteristics. Even after the nucleus of the cell has successfully injected its information into the cytoplasm in preparation for protein synthesis, physiology throws yet another curveball. That final process that converts messenger RNA into protein renders these nascent molecules prey for the proteasome or "cellular garbage disposal." This corkscrew-like structure chews up any protein that isn't carefully shepherded to its final and functional resting place. Like frog larvae gobbled up by a grouper, freshly minted proteins are consumed by the billions before they ever see the light of day.

How, one might ask, does the body ever make anything? Well, the extraordinarily complicated collection of checks and balances built into the system allow only the most important proteins to achieve functional maturity. To regulate the process, cells have synthesized structures known as "heat shock proteins." Their other name is more descriptive—the chaperones. Thus, truly important proteins, recognized by the cell as critical for function, are bearhugged by the chaperones that guide them through the final maturation to adulthood and function. Waiting on the sidelines are enzymes (known as ligases) that, at a moment's notice, pounce upon these newborns and hang residues that send them spinning off to the proteasome for annihilation. It's only by virtue of the chaperone's tenacious grip that needed proteins ever mature.

With these protein structures prepared to assume their function, the icing on the cake is just that. Sugar molecules—in a process called glycosylation—finish the job like lacquer paint on a vintage car.

Now the fun begins. The mature proteins, like recent college grads, have to decide whom they want to date and what they want to wear. For the last billion years or so, the cellular elite has been dominated by phosphate molecules. The transfer of phosphate groups (clusters of phosphorus and oxygen atoms) onto the amino acids serine, threonine, and tyrosine on regulatory proteins throttle the on-off switches of human biology. Whatever it took from epigenetics to small interfering RNAs for these proteins to arrive at their stations, ready for duty, it's the transfer of phosphates that sends the final commands their way.

ESCAPING FROM A LABYRINTH

Any child will tell you that the easiest way to solve a maze is to go to the center and work your way out. The highly convoluted puzzles are fraught with blind alleys and dead ends, making them very confusing when you start from the outside and work in. Yet, this is where our molecular biology colleagues prefer to start. They want to take the 25,000-odd human genes in all their varied forms (splice variants, amplifications, point mutations, SNPs) and solve this human puzzle, top-down.

I, for one, prefer to cheat. Like the child sitting next to you in the restaurant, for whom the kind waitress provided crayons and a worksheet, I go to the center of the maze and work my way out. I freely admit it—I cheat. I get the answer, and then I work my way out, sometimes stopping to talk with a histochemist or a molecular biologist to see if they can characterize what I've already figured out. That's my preferred mode of discovery. Cut to the chase, get the answer, and get out.

It's the medical version of Sutton's Law. His interrogators asked Willy Sutton, a famous bank robber, after his arrest, why he kept robbing banks. He answered, "Because that's where the money is."

So, I rob Mother Nature. I steal the answer, I take it back to my clinic, and I use what works. I'm not looking for a Nobel Prize; I would never expect to get one or any other particular recognition, except one—the good outcome of my patients. I am one of those doctors who really get a kick out of curing patients. My wife often asks me why I can't just practice oncology. But I can't do it. I've seen what laboratory-directed therapy can do, and I can never go back. I can never just be a typical oncologist.

Instead, with my cheating heart, I sneak around the vagaries of human cancer using the most elegant tool of all: human tissue. This extraordinary microcommunity—composed of cells like lymphocytes and histiocytes, stroma, blood vessels, and proteins known as cytokines—represents the ecology of human life. Rather than torturing nuclear DNA until it confesses (however unreliable the data may prove), I peer down upon the totality of cellular response to stress (in this case chemotherapeutics and targeted therapies) to measure how cancer cells will behave. With this global view, the curvature of the horizon becomes clear. The big picture of cell behavior manifests its response to drugs, growth factor withdrawal, and radiation by dying or living to fight another day. The former (cell death) signals a likely clinical response, while the latter indicates likely futile treatment ahead. Skirt those shoals effectively and pilot your patient to safer harbors.

I don't always know why things work. That's the job of PhDs. They will spend a career deciding which amino acid substitution results in a loss of sensitivity to erlotinib in patients with lung cancer. I am quite content to know that erlotinib is the wrong drug. I'll go on to treat 200 patients in the time it takes them to complete their mutational analysis and define but one of the many phenotypes that I observe. I want results and am less concerned with answers.

To get these results, we've pursued functional analytic tests. These laboratory platforms use cellular behavior to define clinical response. Recognizing two fundamental truths, we have been among the first in history to make this work.

The first truth is the realization that cancer largely represents a dysregulation of cell death, not cell growth; cancer doesn't grow too much, it dies too little. Measuring cell death, originally in hematologic malignancies, enabled me to make discoveries that, to this day, remain important clinical therapies. These include chlorodeoxyadenosine for hairy cell leukemia, the curative therapy to this day; and the synergy between purine analogs and alkylating agents, one of the most important treatments for lymphoma. (See Chapter 3.)

But it is the second truth that enabled us to push the envelope of laboratory-directed therapies into solid tumors, those cancers that kill 90 percent of patients. And that truth is the recognition that cancer cells must be maintained in their native state, that the interaction and communication between cells are critical for accurate prediction of response, and that the human tumor microspheroid gently parsed from larger tumor aggregates could serve as my model. These two fundamental principles have made it possible for us to develop the most important treatments for recurrent ovarian cancer and breast cancer and, most recently, to double the survival in lung cancer. However disruptive these simple methodologies may be to our colleagues whose fixation on genomics has turned modern science into little more than pattern recognition, they work and they *must* be applied in the service of cancer patients.

19

Genetic Versus Functional Analysis

Ryan and Michelle could have danced all night. In fact, they almost did. It was New Year's Eve 2010 and everything was going their way.

Ryan Kuper, thirty-eight years old, had moved to Los Angeles a decade earlier to work in the music industry and was now employed by a large insurance company. Despite being very health conscious and a vegetarian, by late January 2011, Ryan couldn't walk up a flight of stairs without stopping halfway to catch his breath. A sudden onset of right-sided chest pain brought him to the emergency room at St. Joseph's Medical Center in Burbank, California, where he was admitted for evaluation of an abnormal chest x-ray.

At this time of year, most people grapple with their new year's resolutions. Not so for Ryan Kuper who now confronted a much more formidable opponent—widely metastatic, poorly differentiated adenocarcinoma of the lung. As a nonsmoker with no significant prior medical history, this all seemed like a bad dream, a dream from which he would awaken at any moment. But it wasn't a dream.

Confirmatory biopsies revealed malignant cells wherever his doctors looked—lung, pleural fluid, pericardium. However well Ryan felt on New Year's Eve 2010, 2011 wasn't sizing up to be a very good year.

The thoracic surgeons placed a catheter into the right chest, allowing Ryan to drain excess fluid every other day to alleviate the shortness of breath caused by pressure in the lung beneath. He was referred to Dr. Raul Mena, an accomplished medical oncologist who practiced in the northern Los Angeles area. Dr. Mena began the process of evaluation and staging in preparation for treatment.

With the advent of the molecular revolution, medical oncologists in 2011 had several new targeted therapies for the treatment of advanced lung cancer. Gefitinib (Iressa) and erlotinib (Tarceva) both target the epidermal growth factor receptor (EGFR). To these agents was added crizotinib, a related kinase inhibitor that has proven active in patients who carry a different mutation known as the ALK gene rearrangement. As a sophisticated medical oncologist, Dr. Mena immediately requested that these tests be completed. A positive result would pave Ryan's way for one or more of these novel treatments, which were only available at that time under clinical trial. Knowing that young, nonsmoking patients with adenocarcinoma were the most likely to carry these genetic abnormalities, Dr. Mena felt cautiously optimistic that Ryan would qualify. Those hopes were dashed when Ryan's mutational analyses all returned "wild type" (no mutations detected). It seemed that Ryan Kuper was just very unlucky.

Scheduled to begin cytotoxic chemotherapy and seeing no easy way out of his dilemma, Ryan, along with his aunt Karlyn, and his father, David, arrived at my office on February 8, 2011. I was puzzled. Virtually all of his tumor markers were normal. He looked the picture of health—slender, tall, and completely at ease with a diagnosis that left me, as an oncologist, cold. My examination revealed diminished breath sounds in the right lung, where a small, sterile plastic tube jutted out of the chest wall. As I finished my examination, I summoned my nurse to assist me as we aspirated 500 milliliters of cloudy yellow fluid from the catheter. Ryan dressed and returned to my office where we discussed his case. Other than an aunt with endometrial cancer, there was no family history of the disease. Ryan's father, a retired urologist, looked troubled as he grasped for an explanation. He explained that Ryan, in his youth, had lived in a bedroom that he had constructed for his son in the basement of their Iowa home.

"Do you think it was radon exposure?" he asked plaintively with a hint of guilt. "It was imponderable," I explained. In point of fact, I really didn't care what had caused the cancer. Ryan Kuper, at thirty-eight years of age, was dying and I needed to do something about it.

To describe the yield of cancer cells from Ryan's lung fluid as plentiful would be an understatement. The pleural effusion was chockablock full of cancer cells—big, juicy, cohesive, mucinous adenocarcinoma cells were everywhere we looked under the microscope. We set up assays for every drug and combination we could think of, as well as every targeted therapy. With the completion of the analysis, there was one finding that stuck out. Ryan was sensitive to crizotinib, very sensitive. But without the right gene mutation, he couldn't get it. I called Dr. Mena to confirm that the ALK gene rearrangement was negative. "Absolutely," he said.

I had no such misgivings regarding the accuracy of the EGFR tests, as both Iressa and Tarceva were clearly inactive in vitro. But the crizotinib results stuck in my craw. I called Ryan and asked if he would provide us additional fluid following his next catheter drainage. We repeated the test. Again, crizotinib was active. I contacted Dr. Mark G. Kris at the Memorial Sloan-Kettering Cancer Center in New York. I wondered whether the results for crizotinib might reflect a different mutation, c-MET. Dr. Kris kindly referred me to Dr. Edward B. Garon at UCLA who offered to run additional molecular analyses on the sample. I then contacted Dr. Sai-Hong Ignatius Ou, a member of the faculty at the University of California, Irvine. As one of the authors on the original *New England Journal of Medicine* paper that described the use of crizotinib on ALK gene mutation patients, Dr. Ou had access to crizotinib—a drug that had not yet been approved by the FDA. Might he possibly be able to accrue Ryan to a crizotinib trial? The answer was no. Without the appropriate ALK gene mutation, Ryan was just plain out of luck.

I felt stymied, claustrophobic, and desperate. Ryan, for all the world, looked like someone who would respond to crizotinib, and I couldn't get it. I corresponded regularly with Ryan and explained that I would continue to work to find the drug. Alas, there was no source. Not here, not in Europe, Japan, Korea, or China. Nowhere. It reminded me of my earliest work with Iressa, a drug that was approved in Europe and Japan before it was approved in the United States. More than once I had dispatched family members to Tokyo to procure Iressa for their relatives here in the United States who had been found sensitive in vitro at a time when the drug was not yet FDA approved for use. They would return and provide this life-saving therapy to their family members, predicated on our results. But there was no source of crizotinib—none. And then, it occurred to me. There are no perfect tests. Every analysis has error bars, and the ALK gene rearrangement tests were still being worked out. Maybe, just maybe, Ryan's results were wrong. I needed confirmation. I got back in touch with Dr. Ou and learned that tissue remained from Ryan's original biopsy. Through his connections, we were able to bypass the usual referral networks and send the tissue sample directly to the Massachusetts General Hospital, a recognized reference laboratory skilled in these analyses. As Ryan's clinical condition deteriorated, I conferred with his medical oncologist in Burbank and recommended that we begin cisplatin plus gemcitabine, the most active regimen I could find.

With a couple of cycles of therapy under his belt, Ryan felt a little better. The fluid accumulation slowed and he gained a little weight. I awaited Dr. Ou's results with bated breath. And then it came. Ryan was ALK gene positive. His original laboratory analyses were incorrect. Our perseverance paid off. He could now qualify for crizotinib. At his next follow-up visit with Dr. Ou, he began therapy and responded almost immediately. Now, as we approach the one-year mark, Ryan is back at work full-time and enjoying his life on two pills a day. He has had no side effects.

The saga of Ryan Kuper is instructive on numerous levels. First, he is an example of the new era of therapies that work well on a select few patients with the right type of cancer. Second, he exemplifies the need for a patient advocate: a doctor or family member who will not take no for an answer. I would not let go of Ryan Kuper. I knew there was a way out and I was going to find it. Finally, Ryan's story is among the best examples of the predictive validity of human tumor primary culture analyses. My results repeated over and over didn't lie. Ryan was sensitive to crizotinib, Ryan needed crizotinib, and Ryan was going to get crizotinib. His molecular profile notwithstanding, Ryan got the drug he needed and lives to fight another day. For me, it is a gratifying example of the power of functional analysis and reinforces my belief that physiology trumps informatics.

Modern oncologists are enamored with molecular biology. Using DNA analyses they will apply the results to select treatments that would otherwise seem improbable if not absurd. Blinded by science, they luxuriate in the new discipline of genomic profiling, yet lack the scientific experience to examine the legitimate applications of these high-tech platforms. Leaving behind their insights, experience, and clinical acumen, they are misled by their brethren in the field of genetic analysis.

This all reminds me of a joke my mother once told me. A grandmother, pushing a carriage carrying two cute grandchildren, is approached by an admiring bystander. The woman congratulates the grandmother on these lovely children. "Yes," says the grandmother, beaming with pride. "They are very cute. But you should see the photographs."

20

Targeted Therapies

If there is one theme in this book that stands out above all others, it is the repeated mantra that *cancer doesn't grow too much, it dies too little.* I would be so bold as to say that *every* therapy that works, works by killing cells. From radiation to hormones to cytotoxic chemotherapy, patients only respond when their cancer cells die. If this were true for conventional therapies, would it carry over to the new classes of targeted drugs?

The term "targeted therapy" arose in the last decade to describe drugs that selectively "target" features that are unique to cancer populations. Many of these drugs act upon the cellular communication networks known as signal transduction pathways. Among the most commonly studied pathways are those associated with cell surface proteins known as receptors. The epidermal *growth* factor receptor (EGFR) and the insulin-like *growth* factor receptor (IGFR) are frequent targets.

Growth? I began to wonder whether the operative term "growth" was being used correctly. Was it "growth" in the truest sense of the term or the absence of death in cell populations that were "growing" at a normal rate that caused tumors to expand? After all, the people who named these growth factors were educated in an era when cancer was viewed as a disease of cell growth. To their way of thinking, the cancer's success was predicated on its growth, and it followed that cancer-causing mutations must enhance growth. It all fit together so nicely.

However, just as America was named for the explorer Amerigo Vespucci, growth factors were named by investigators whose world-view of cancer causation could only see one explanation for the disease—cell growth. This became abundantly clear in 2000, when I had the opportunity to examine the most prominent solid-tumor-targeted agent of that time, AZD1839 (gefitinib, later known as Iressa).

This small molecule, known as a tyrosine kinase inhibitor, works by blocking the chemical signal that occurs following the activation of the EGFR. It was developed based upon its potent "growth inhibitory" effects in cell lines. We were kindly provided a small quantity of the drug to study several years before clinical trials were reported.

I remember my senior technician Craig Chow coming to me in 2001 and explaining, contrary to expectations, that the drug was killing cells in our primary cultures. I examined his data to be sure that the correct controls with DMSO (the solvent for the gefitinib) had been conducted. To my surprise, his data was pristine. I could find no artifacts. We continued our studies and with the completion of 87 analyses submitted our findings to the American Association for Cancer Research (AACR) meeting in late 2001 (Nagourney 2002).

With the acceptance of the abstract, I was invited to the special symposium on gefitinib held that year at the AACR meeting. The participants were intrigued by my observations, particularly when I suggested that adenocarcinoma of the lung would be the best target for the drug. It wasn't until months later at the American Society of Clinical Oncology meeting and the report on the IDEAL I and II clinical trials that my findings were confirmed. Gefitinib moved rapidly through FDA approval, followed thereafter by the closely related erlotinib (Tarceva). The field of solid–tumor targeted therapy was born.

The following year, I reported our follow-up results in which we examined not only the activity, but also the combination of gefitinib with other drugs. This time we found that gefitinib did not favorably interact with cisplatin, suggesting that this recently approved targeted lung cancer drug and the most widely used conventional chemotherapy drug for this disease would not have a happy marriage. Unfortunately, the senior investigators at neither AstraZeneca nor Genentech listened. They went on to conduct four large, and entirely negative, clinical trials in which patients with advanced lung cancer were given Iressa plus carboplatin and Taxol, or Iressa plus cisplatin and gemcitabine (the INTACT I and INTACT II trials). Both studies were abject failures and AstraZeneca's flagship drug appeared to be on thin ice.

Unfazed, Genentech sponsored virtually the exact same trials (TALENT and TRIBUTE), substituting their targeted agent Tarceva for Iressa. Once again, the random combination of a targeted agent and a conventional chemotherapy combination for lung cancer proved ineffective. Targeted therapy had suffered its first big hiccup.

How might one explain my laboratory's ability, using cell death, to accurately predict the clinical efficacy of so-called growth inhibitors? After all, we weren't growing cells. The answer was simple. These were not growth inhibitors. I reasoned that exposure to epidermal growth factor provided cells a survival advantage—not a growth advantage. These epidermal growth factor (EGF)–driven cancers were not being driven to grow, but encouraged to remain alive. Epidermal growth factor wasn't a growth factor at all. I began to call it "epidermal antideath factor." And the small quantities of EGF circulating in the bloodstream were the drip-irrigation of cell maintenance. To test this hypothesis scientifically, I reasoned that common downstream signals could be identified for these survival pathways. Following the publication of a paper in the *Journal of Biological Chemistry* in 2002, I began to compare the EGFR tyrosine kinase inhibitors (gefitinib and erlotinib) with agents that were associated with other survival signals. We started with the small molecule wortmannin that blocks the survival signals associated with insulin. Again, we saw cell death in the test tube. When we then exposed cancer cells to wortmannin and gefitinib—both alone and together—we saw a strong relationship between their actions and evidence of potent combination effects known as synergy. The analysis of our data, subsequently reported at the 2003 AACR meeting, confirmed that these so-called growth factors were, in fact, survival factors.

This all fit very neatly with the elegant phrase coined by Dr. I. Bernard Weinstein at Columbia University, who described cancer cells with mutations in these pathways as "oncogene addicted." Once these cells got hooked on the particular survival pathway, they couldn't live without it. Like a drug addict deprived of his heroin, these cancer cells, when exposed to gefitinib or erlotinib, went through the most severe form of withdrawal—death.

It was perfect. It was exactly what we were seeing in the laboratory. These cells were addicted to the growth factor pathway, and we were administering the antidote. Unlike the drug addict who suddenly roars out of his stupor following a dose of Narcan (the drug used by emergency room physicians to reverse the effects of a heroin overdose), these hyped-up cancer cells dropped dead. The whole process only took three days, and it was every bit as easy to measure the effect of targeted therapies in our laboratory as it was to measure the effects of conventional chemotherapy drugs. If it is said that "all roads lead to Rome," then we were now certain that all effective cancer therapies lead to cell death.

Just as Christopher Columbus believed that he had discovered a new route to India, cancer researchers were convinced that they had discovered growth factors. With the recognition that targeted drugs worked by interrupting survival pathways, I was now absolutely convinced that we could apply our platform to accelerate the discovery and application of effective targeted therapies.

WHAT'S GOOD FOR THE GOOSE IS GOOD FOR THE GANDER

Might it be that all of the targeted therapies were working through related survival signals? If we had shown that the EGFR and IGF signals were survival signals, then there would be reason to believe that the advantages utilized by tumors with various mutations were ultimately survival advantages as well.

With this in mind, we expanded the scope of our investigation to include virtually every known small molecule inhibitor for a signal pathway. From PI3K to HER2, from mTOR to AKT, from MEK/ERK to c-MET, from sonic hedgehog to notch, and from PKC to EML4-ALK, all of these pathways seemed to function through cell survival. Regardless of the complexity of the pathway (or its name), I and my laboratory staff became only further convinced that cancer is a disease of altered cell survival. Recognizing this has enabled me to pursue the rational combination of signal inhibitors and has confirmed my growing belief that intelligent combinations of these therapies will have a meaningful impact on patient outcomes in the near future.

A PERFECT EXAMPLE OF OUTLIVING CANCER—SUE ALLEN

One afternoon I was working in my laboratory and received a call from G. Nathan Newman, MD, a primary care physician who spoke slowly and with a great deal of emotional distress. "I have a patient I'd like you to see right away. She's sitting in my office with her husband, and it looks like she has widely metastatic lung cancer. She's forty-four years old."

I told him to send her immediately.

As the patient was traveling to my office, Dr. Newman called me back and said, "I was afraid to speak candidly with them in the room, but this looks as bad as it gets." I felt the discomfort in his voice as he said, "She could be my wife."

Minutes later, a perky, pretty young woman with a tall, strapping husband in tow, arrived at my laboratory. Sue had a cute way of talking, pursing her lips at the end of each statement with a catlike smile. Her husband, a fireman and emergency medical technician, was only too familiar with the implications of metastatic lung cancer. Sue, herself a nurse in the neonatal intensive care unit, was no stranger to serious illness, and I could see in her eyes a tearful look of terror.

I explained what I did and how I did it, and that I would very gladly enroll her in a clinical trial that we were conducting in lung cancer. The study was designed to use our laboratory platform to match patients to chemotherapy drugs. In order to participate, Sue would need a biopsy. A CT scan revealed obvious disease located on the lung and central portion of the chest (known as the mediastinum), but it appeared that she would require a surgical biopsy of the lung as well. Contemplating the invasive nature of the procedure, I suggested to Sue and her husband that she might wish to obtain additional opinions. After all, there was no guarantee that my recommendations would work.

Within a short distance of my office, there are many experts in lung cancer management. Despite my deep-seated belief that I could help her, and my desire to do so, I personally called Ronald B. Natale, MD, at the Cedars-Sinai Medical Center in Los Angeles and arranged an appointment for several days hence. Dr. Natale provided an excellent consultation and recommended a very reasonable combination of chemotherapeutics. Sue and her husband considered the options and decided to return to Long Beach to participate in our study.

Days later, another PET/CT was conducted that revealed new areas of disease, including a large cluster of lymph nodes at the base of the right neck. The bad news was that the disease was on the move. The good news was that I could now biopsy the neck to get a sample.

Within days the results were in hand. Sue had a perfect profile of response to the new class of drugs known as epidermal growth factor tyrosine kinase inhibitors. Iressa had been approved the year earlier and Tarceva was just approved. In keeping with the results of the analysis, I proceeded to place Sue on first-line Tarceva.

In 2004, absolutely no one used Tarceva first-line. The genetic mutations that would later guide the selection of this class of drugs would not be reported in the literature by investigators at Memorial Sloan-Kettering Cancer Center and Dana-Farber Cancer Institute for another year. No laboratories were offering these predictive tests. The only thing I had to go on was her sensitivity to Tarceva in vitro. At the time, the standard of care was platinum-based doublets—carboplatin plus Taxol, cisplatin plus gemcitabine, cisplatin plus navelbine—that's what everyone got. That's what I was expecting to give Sue. That's what Dr. Natale recommended. But I couldn't. The laboratory identified Tarceva and I felt duty-bound to give it.

I agonized over what to do. I wanted to give her this unusual treatment, but it was so far out. So I called Sue and her husband and I invited them to the laboratory. I took them into my slide-reading room and sat each of them at the multiheaded microscope. I showed them the plump, purple, grapelike clusters of cancer cells from the tissue culture analysis. "This is your cancer," I said. And, changing the slides, "This is your cancer on drugs." The dose response curves were perfect. At each concentration there were zero living cells. I felt sure that Sue would respond to a pill a day. I just knew it. But would she agree to take it? Sue and her husband looked at the slides, looked at each other, and said, "Let's go for it."

To describe her response to this therapy as dramatic would be an understatement. Sue turned on a dime. The lymph nodes in her neck disappeared. The cough disappeared. So did the shortness of breath. A few months later, her CT scan was remarkably improved. A few months after that, it was normal. Sue was in remission on a pill a day. She had never received chemotherapy. We had our first experience with laboratory-directed targeted therapy and it worked.

About a year after Sue had begun treatment and while she was enjoying an excellent remission, investigators published the results of their analyses identifying a mutation in the EGFR gene that conferred sensitivity to Tarceva. I identified a laboratory at the City of Hope that was offering this study for about $1,000 and submitted her tissue blocks for analysis. Convinced that she would carry the mutation, I awaited the results with anticipation.

To my surprise, Sue was found to carry a novel deletion in the region of the EGFR gene that was not associated with sensitivity to Tarceva. The written report suggested that this finding did not support the use of Tarceva in this patient. Here was Sue, a full year in remission on a drug that the genetic analysis recommended against. Not only had we shown that the functional platform could identify patients before the gene mutations were known to exist, but it was able to identify heretofore unrecognized variants undetected by the available gene tests. Sue was entering her second year of remission on a treatment no one else would have given her.

During the second year of her remission, a mild elevation in Sue's CEA (a tumor marker) blood test led to a formal reevaluation with PET/CT. This identified re-growth of disease at the center of the chest. The options were to treat with chemotherapy or rebiopsy. We opted for the latter and Sue underwent a minithoracotomy to procure tissue. While all other areas of disease remained in good control, Sue now had growth of a more resistant population for which Tarceva had lost its effect. Despite this setback, her new profile for the combination of cisplatin plus gemcitabine was a perfect match. Recognizing that most of her disease remained under good control, we added cisplatin plus gemcitabine, and Sue entered her second remission.

Over the ensuing two years, Sue's PET/CT scans revealed minor changes in her disease, which led me to introduce increasingly novel treatments. First, I added hydroxychloroquine. This antiparasitic agent (also used in autoimmune diseases like lupus) had been shown in a laboratory model to overcome Tarceva resistance. Indeed, on this novel combination, her disease again stabilized. However, by the fourth year a new area of PET/CT uptake was found in the left lung and continued to progress despite my best ministrations. I had no alternative but to resect this area to study its behavior, and a surgical procedure was scheduled.

The findings were unexpected. While every one of Sue's prior cancer biopsies had revealed adenocarcinoma, this new area of disease was squamous cell carcinoma. Sue had an entirely new lung cancer! We opted to use local radiation therapy. Sue completed her treatment without undue toxicity and remained well for the better part of an additional year.

Sue never let her cancer get in the way of her life. She traveled to Hawaii, accompanied her husband on ski trips in the Sierras, and attended to the needs of her eight-year-old son. More often than not, when I would ask Sue to join me at a symposium or participate in an interview, she would decline because she was in the Sacramento area working on her walnut farm or skiing at Mammoth Mountain.

It was during just such a trip that Sue, an accomplished skier, stumbled off the chairlift, dragging her left leg. The next day an MRI revealed metastatic disease that had spread to the base of the brain, an area known as the cerebellum.

On January 10, 2010, Barry Ceverha, MD, performed a craniotomy and resected a large, metastatic lesion from the brain. Our analysis, conducted upon the tissue submitted to the laboratory, revealed a surprising finding. In retrospect, perhaps it shouldn't have been so surprising. The drug response profiles were virtually superimposable upon those done in the original study nearly five years earlier. This tumor, freshly removed from Sue's brain, was identical to that tumor that I had removed from her right neck at the time of the original biopsy. As I considered the finding, it became increasingly clear why. Of course it's the same, I realized. These cancer cells had hidden behind the blood-brain barrier (a vascular defense that separates the brain from the rest of the body) since Sue was originally diagnosed in 2004. They lived in what we call in cancer medicine a "sanctuary site." They hadn't traveled to the brain in the last few years, but instead they had been there all along. That is why these cells had no previous exposure to the chemotherapy drugs, which had worked so well for her earlier treatment. This suggested that the tumors were chemotherapeutic virgins and, I reasoned, should respond very well to radiation that mimics the effect of drugs like cisplatin. Unfortunately, these chemo-naïve cells gave me no insight into the best treatment for the tumors that continued to progress in the rest of Sue's body.

This was old news. I needed new treatments.

Sue received CyberKnife radiation therapy to the brain followed by the placement of metal markers (known as fiducials) used to guide further CyberKnife radiation to areas of the lung and mediastinum. With all of the time it took to prepare and treat Sue, I had all but lost touch with her. With each passing course of radiation, a new area of disease would crop up. Further radiation, more disease. Finally, Sue called me and said that she could no longer swallow.

A CT scan revealed a giant lymph node in the right central chest compressing her esophagus. The gastroenterologist could not pass through an endoscope, and for that reason no dilation could be done. Sue couldn't eat. She couldn't even swallow. She was deteriorating rapidly. The radiation therapists felt the site was too large and too close to vital structures for further radiation. We decided to biopsy Sue's tumor, yet again.

Sue was living on Ensure and losing weight at an alarming rate. She found it so difficult to swallow that she often needed to spit up her own saliva. The biopsy was conducted and the results proved extremely instructive. After all the drugs and treatments Sue had received, the tumor had clocked around to an entirely new profile of sensitivity. The most favorable combination—navelbine plus irinotecan plus 5-FU—was not a combination I had ever used in lung cancer. Nor, for that matter, had anyone else. While I would've preferred to use the oral formulation of 5-FU known as Xeloda to IV infusions, Sue couldn't swallow, so we moved forward with the intravenous formulation.

Therapy began immediately and, just as quickly, Sue got better.

Her elevated CEA blood levels fell to normal. The gagging and difficulty swallowing disappeared. She began to eat normally and regained her weight. She and her family returned to their normal busy schedules. Sue was back. Christmas 2010 was a celebration.

Then, in early January 2011, a repeat PET/CT revealed an unexpected finding. While most of the previously identified areas in the lung had completely resolved, the left upper lobe of the left lung had completely collapsed. An obstruction in the main airway of the left lung blocked all air entry. Emergency consultation with Septimiu Dan Murgu, MD, an interventional pulmonologist at the University of California, Irvine, was obtained in hope that a stent or laser procedure would open the left lung. But this was not the case. Biopsies were obtained and—lo and behold—an entirely new profile of drug sensitivity was identified. Sue's tumor, for the first time, was sensitive to Taxol.

Despite prior exposure to radiation, and following careful consultation with the radiation oncologist, we opted to use CyberKnife to open up the area of obstruction in the left lung. Sue responded immediately. With Dr. Murgu's expertise, we were able to maintain aeration of the left lung and return Sue, yet again, to normal activities. The next chapter in her chemotherapeutic management with Taxol-based therapy was about to begin.

Substituting Taxol for navelbine, Sue continued on a three-drug combination of Taxol, irinotecan, and Xeloda. With the resolution of Sue's previous swallowing difficulties, we were able to prescribe the oral formulation Xeloda that I had originally hoped to use. Once again, Sue responded. There was no reocclusion of the left lung, the tumor markers remained under perfect control, and Sue returned to her life.

Over the 2011 Thanksgiving weekend, I received a voicemail at my laboratory. It was Sue Allen leaving a message of heartfelt thanks. Calling from Northern California where she was spending the holiday with her family, she said how grateful she was for all we had done for her.

Despite the rigors of Sue's history, she has lived what would have to be considered a virtually normal life for approaching seven years. She has raised a young child to the edge of his teen years and has enjoyed a very active lifestyle. I have no intention of giving up on Sue and, I assure you, she has no intention of quitting.

Our most recent conversation with Sue Allen was late July 2012 as she and her family were preparing for a three-week vacation in Montana.

2 1

The Future of Cancer Research Lies Behind Us

In the southeastern Pacific Ocean lies Easter Island, also known as Rapa Nui. It was here that a small molecule, rapamycin (sirolimus), was isolated from a streptomyces broth. Under development by Wyeth Pharmaceuticals, the compound known as Rapamune gained broad use as an immunosuppressant in patients undergoing organ transplantation. As scientists examined this compound's mode of action, they recognized its impact upon a protein contained within the cell responsible for the regulation of a number of metabolic processes. As it was the compound rapamycin that enabled these investigators to discover the protein, they named this metabolic intermediate "mammalian target of rapamycin" (mTOR).

With each passing year, researchers delved deeper into the role of mTOR in human biology, ultimately recognizing it as a fundamental linchpin for cellular response to environmental stress. We now recognize that mTOR sits at the crossroads of insulin signaling in cells and regulates cell size and cell proliferation. By inhibiting this protein, the human lymphocytes that respond to foreign antigens, such as those associated with a transplanted donor kidney, could be shut down to prevent kidney rejection. What became more interesting over time was the growing recognition of this pathway's importance in all of cellular biology, including cancer. Today, a number of commercial products, including temsirolimus and everolimus—inhibitors of the mTOR pathway—are being used for the treatment of cancers that range from lymphoma to breast cancer to kidney cancer. Interestingly, these anticancer agents function by inhibiting metabolic pathways that regulate protein synthesis and glucose metabolism.

More interesting still is the fact that rapamycin isolated from a bacterial broth is, in the truest sense of the word, a targeted therapy. Yet, rapamycin is not a product of the human genome project. Rapamycin just is. It is, because organisms, long before the first scientist was ever born, needed protection. Protection from one another and protection from other predatory organisms, and they utilized products like rapamycin to defend themselves.

What, after all, is the most effective defense at the level of a cell or multicellular organism? Placed in harm's way, do you confront your aggressor with birth control or a lethal weapon? Clearly, primordial organisms recognized that the death of the offending entity needed to be quick. It wasn't enough to prevent the bacteria, fungi, or algae from reproducing. Instead, a swift death could best be achieved by unhinging the most fundamental underpinning of life itself—cellular metabolism. It is not surprising that many natural products induce lethal injury to cells at the level of metabolism.

Long before humankind discovered DNA, tribal shamans used metabolic toxins to treat diseases, even cancers. It is only now, after our five-decade foray into genomics, that we are rediscovering metabolic medicine. Behind every new genomic discovery there lies a deep-seated connection to energy production and utilization. It is not surprising that the cell jealously guards its most critical metabolic pathways. Attempts to utilize metabolic poisons are fraught with hazards. There is no cell in the human body that can exist without the well-oiled machinery of energy production. These biochemical processes with names like glycolysis, the urea cycle, the pentose shunt, and the Krebs cycle are wheels within wheels of energy-producing gears. Each of the cogs in these gears is a small-molecule metabolic intermediate. The tiniest alteration in just one cog can bring the entire machine to a halt.

I have often said that cancer is easy to cure. I have no doubt that I can stop any cancer dead in its tracks. The problem is that the patient can't possibly survive the therapy.

Investigators like Otto Warburg and Albert Szent-Györgyi in decades past recognized the role of electron transport in cellular energy production, most of which occurs at the level of the mitochondrion. The metabolism of foodstuffs—principally glucose—ultimately yields a reservoir of energy-containing molecules known as adenosine triphosphate (ATP). Every chemical reaction in the body then taps into this reservoir of energy to maintain the processes we know as life. For generations, scientists have recognized that substances capable of inhibiting the production of ATP, such as rotenone, amytal, antimycin A, and cyanide, are poisons because they turn off ATP production at different points. For obvious reasons, substances like cyanide have never been used as therapies. Yet, with our growing recognition of cellular metabolism as a target for therapy, certain toxins have resurfaced as potential therapies. Arsenic trioxide, now widely used in the treatment of certain forms of leukemia, is just such a metabolic poison. Arsenic (atomic number 33), with its atomic structure close to that of its neighbor phosphorus (atomic number 15), can sneak in and replace phosphorus in its critical role in energy production and storage. This can grind critical metabolic processes to a halt. Interestingly, microorganisms isolated from Mono Lake in California have recently been reported to use arsenic in place of phosphorus in their metabolic processes. While we await confirmation of this finding, it represents a fundamental departure from much of what we have been taught in biochemistry.

As the complexities of human metabolism are examined through the lens of modern scientific technology, we find that cancer research is undergoing not a revolution, but an evolution. An evolution predicated on greater technical skill applied to the same age-old questions. Where biochemists of yesteryear labored to adjust the conditions of their chemical reactions to analyze the role of enzymes at the level of stoichiometry (the study of concentration and quantities of chemical reaction outcomes), today we have high throughput machines with names like the Seahorse XF Extracellular Flux Analyzer that examine the same processes in a microsecond. The science hasn't changed, just the technology.

From the 1990s into the new millennium we have witnessed the birth of targeted therapies. The targets of these therapeutic agents have been identified through the genomic analysis of signaling pathways in cancers. As the malignantly transformed cells hijack these pathways to their advantage, they inadvertently open themselves up to the effects of pathway inhibitors. Drugs with names like erlotinib, sunitinib, and crizotinib disrupt cellular circuitry and dampen the survival signals responsible for malignant transformation. To our disappointment, the sometimes dramatic responses to these agents are usually short-lived. Evolution occurs at every level and every cancer cell deprived of its survival signal by a small molecule will do its best to circumvent that inhibition. The dramatic responses in melanoma to the newest member of the class vemurafenib (a drug that targets the signaling pathway BRAF) are almost always followed by the rapid regrowth of vemurafenib-resistant tumors.

Why? The answer lies in the realization that these circuits are several layers removed from the most important aspect of cancer survival—cellular metabolism. The real action is at the level of the mitochondria where all of the energy that drives the circuits is produced. Like an enemy's nuclear facility, the cell guards its most fundamental processes in hardened bunkers. In its own way, the cancer cell teases the medical oncology community with its own version of the taunt "You can have the secret to energy production when you peel cancer's cold dead fingers off its mitochondria."

22

The Causes of Cancer

Much of this book has focused on the treatment of advanced cancers. That is, patients for whom available treatments had failed, or those for whom no known treatment existed. Yet, these same patients went on to achieve durable benefits based upon the results of our laboratory analyses. The drugs and combinations we identified for these individuals worked because they reactivated the process of programmed cell death and caused the cancer cells to regress. But, how do cancer cells go wrong in the first place and why?

In chapter 6 we began the discussion of apoptosis and touched upon viral oncogenesis (causes of cancer) and mentioned the now well-established association between human papilloma virus (HPV) and cancers of the cervix and oral cavity. While it's hard to applaud viruses in their assault on the human body, one cannot deny the elegance of their deception. After all, these organisms selectively, specifically, and highly effectively disarm the most sophisticated defenses of the human cell in service of their own reproduction. Here, the adversarial relationship between host and pathogen hinges upon a few select targets that start the ball rolling from viral infection to malignant transformation. But what of the myriad of other events that lead to cancer? To our knowledge only a minority of cancers are caused by viruses. So then, what drives the other 80 or 90 percent of these diseases?

151

Not surprisingly, every cancer-causing event must, at some point, disarm the process of programmed cell death. After all, every cell is hardwired to commit suicide if a mutation is detected. Viruses, by inserting their own genetic material into the cell's DNA, create an abnormality that the cell perceives as a mutation. In response to these forms of damage, cells develop defenses. The two most important of these are p53 and retinoblastoma protein. The products of these genes conduct surveillance and monitor the integrity of human chromosomes. The detection of a mutation—or viral DNA sequence—causes these proteins to stop the cell in its tracks and forces the cell to do one of two things.

The first is to repair the damage, remove the mutation, or reject the virus. Failing this, these same proteins initiate the process of programmed cell death. The dictum of p53 and retinoblastoma is "straighten up and fly right" or don't fly at all. Not surprisingly, viruses have evolved to evade the effects of p53 and retinoblastoma. Proteins then bind to and inactivate these cellular crossing guards, thereby allowing the viruses free access to the cell's reproductive machinery.

In the absence of viruses, these same proteins can be knocked out by mutation. Ironically, these mutations occur within the very genes that code for the proteins designed to respond to mutations. Terms like SNP (single nucleotide polymorphisms) deletion, missense, frame shift, and splice variant describe but a few of the genetic changes found in cancers. Regardless of the specific change in DNA code, the result is to allow these damaged and otherwise programmed-to-die cells to survive and propagate.

In the absence of viruses, how would these spontaneous mutations arise?

The normal human cell is a veritable factory of cancer-causing chemicals known as free radicals. These toxic forms of oxygen spin off 5 percent of all mitochondrial energy production (oxidative phosphorylation) and spill into the cellular cytoplasm, mostly in the form of superoxide. Free radical oxygen damages cell membranes and can break or cross-link the genetic material that makes up chromosomes. Anything that increases the production of these oxygen radicals can increase mutation and cancer. Why, one might ask, would the body allow these toxic substances to exist within the cell? In part, it is because cellular metabolism is so high in energy that these byproducts cannot be avoided. However, many normal human reactions depend upon free radical activity. Among them, the white cells (known as polymorphonuclear [PMN] leukocytes) intentionally release free radical oxygen to kill bacteria. Sites of infection and inflammation are not surprisingly hot beds of free radical activity. It is now recognized that the tumor microenvironment contains large numbers of inflammatory cells, and these immune cells participate in the process of carcinogenesis. Inflammation, a critical component of injury and wound healing, is fertile ground for cancer. In fact, cancer has been described as "the wound that will not heal."

We have long recognized that environmental factors contribute to cancer. Many of the substances found in cigarette smoke and barbecued foods are free radical chemicals. In addition, the metabolic breakdown of certain forms of food during digestion can produce free radicals. Trans fatty acids are shunted off to a small intracellular organelle known as the peroxisome where they undergo chemical degradation by enzymes known as peroxidases. These enzymes, in turn, spin off molecules of hydrogen peroxide that can go on to damage the cell and create mutations.

Concerns surrounding electromagnetic radiation and cell phones reflect yet another possible mechanism of carcinogenesis—the transfer of microwave energy to human tissues. While the exact mechanisms continue to be studied, the generation of heat and direct energy transfer known as the piezoelectric effect may be causally related.

Among the most potent pathways in humans are those associated with the steroid hormones. These include estrogen, progesterone, and testosterone. As these chemicals circulate throughout the body, they arrive at cells of interest where they activate growth and survival in those cells that carry specific proteins known as receptors. The genes that code for these receptors are part of an extraordinary network known as the steroid super gene family. So potent are these genetic elements that they influence every aspect of human existence—from body height and weight to the function of the neurons in our brains. Steroid hormones are chemical derivatives of the molecule cholesterol, differing only in the placement of a few oxygen, hydrogen, and double bonds. Their unique structure enables them to bind and activate the specific pathway for which they are designed: testosterone to the androgen receptor, estradiol to the estrogen receptor, and so forth. The location and distance between these oxygen and hydrogen atoms on the steroid molecule dictate which receptor they will activate.

Some years ago, synthetic chemists realized they could mimic these effects by synthesizing chemically distinct but structurally similar molecules. Among the most potent and famous of these substances is diethylstilbestrol (DES). While this molecule—a stilbene—looks nothing like estradiol, it potently activates all of the same pathways associated with estrogen. This "bio-mimicry," heralded as a breakthrough for therapeutics, has now returned to haunt us in an environment riddled with hormonelike substances known as xenoestrogens.

Sophisticated petrochemistry uses crude oil to synthesize the medicines, synthetic fibers, and plastics that have so influenced modern existence. Despite the many advances, modern man now finds himself swimming in a sea of carcinogens of his own making. These environmental contaminants bludgeon the body's delicate balances, overdriving the tissues of the breast and uterus in women and the prostate in men—ultimately resulting in cancer.

While steroid hormones influence innumerable biological processes, they do one thing particularly well—keep cells alive. And as we've noted many times before, in multicellular organisms the most dangerous cell of all is the cell that refuses to die. During our reproductive years, normal levels of steroid hormones maintain our capacity for propagation. Continued exposure to these substances provides the "drip-irrigation" that sponsors abnormal clones and leads to cancer. Whether it is estrogen supplements taken by post-menopausal women or chronic exposure to xenoestrogens, long-lived cells provide a reservoir for malignant transformation.

Within each cell are cascades of critical regulatory proteins with names like RAS and RAF (the most common and potent gain-of-function cancer mutations). There are also signaling pathways known as insulin-like growth factors, closely related to the protein hormones used by the body to regulate cellular uptake of nutrients, like amino acids and glucose. When mutations occur in these critical proteins, the common thread is cell survival. These mutations, however simple or complex, must at some point disarm the natural process of programmed cell death and enable these dysfunctional cells to remain alive, contrary to the most profound dictates of multicellular existence. John Lennon said, "Life is what happens to you while you're busy making other plans." I would add that cancer is what happens while you're busy activating other pathways.

In science, we use the terms "lumpers" and "splitters" to describe researchers who seek commonality (lumpers) or differences (splitters) in their respective disciplines. Based on our discussion in this chapter, cancer as a disease would appear to belong within the purview of the lumpers. Despite this, virtually all research dollars today go to support the work of the splitters. For decades, the term "cancer" was used generically to describe all malignancies. Cancer researchers then increasingly defined distinctions between tumor types, and cancer research became progressively more siloed. Lung cancer physicians worked only on lung cancer, while entire societies developed to study breast cancer, ovarian cancer, and other subtypes. It became increasingly common to speak of cancer not as one disease, but many, perhaps hundreds. Yet, this meandering baseline will soon return to the view that cancer is but one disease, as we realize that cancer is not one mutation or another, but instead a fundamental change in cellular metabolism that results from a wide variety of genetic changes.

There is a commonality to biological existence. Autotrophs, like photosynthetic plants, use the same intermediates (NAD, ATP) in the production of sugar that heterotrophs like humans use to consume sugars. Musicians use the same notes to play Chopin and the Rolling Stones. It is not the notes, but how they're played that determines the sound. Cancer and normal biology share the same metabolic processes. It is the goal of cancer research to define the nuances that distinguish the benign from the malignant state.

23

To Cancer and Beyond

In the spring of 1921, Dr. Frederick Banting, physician and lecturer in pharmacology at the University of Toronto, approached Dr. J. J. R. Macleod, professor of physiology at the university, to ask if he could have access to the professor's laboratories to pursue his interests in pancreatic hormones. Dr. Macleod agreed and supplied him Charles Best—a medical student at the University—as an assistant.

Together, Best and Banting conducted experiments on dogs to identify the islets of Langerhans (small collections of cells found within the human pancreas) as the source of insulin. This discovery led to many awards, including the Nobel Prize in physiology in 1923. This breakthrough would never have been made had it not been for the disease diabetes mellitus. Diabetes mellitus, one of the most common endocrinological disorders, is characterized by hyperglycemia (elevated blood sugars). The condition leads to the predisposition for cardiac disease, stroke, life-threatening infections, peripheral vascular disease, neuropathy, and, in the untreated state—death.

Disease states are windows on human biology, and it is only through the disease states that normal physiology can be explored.

Cancer is just such a window on human biology.

SPLITTERS AND LUMPERS

It is through the study of cancer that we will someday understand
aging, dementia, autoimmunity, atherosclerosis, arthritis, obesity,
congenital disorders, degenerative diseases, and death. Cancer
arises from the dysregulation of cellular death signals and comman-
deers cellular survival signals to the detriment of the organism as
a whole. Throughout this book we have referred to cancer as a disease of cell death, a disease in which mutated and damaged cells
fail to die on schedule. In so doing, these errant cells disrupt the
carefully orchestrated symphony of functions we recognize as multicellular existence. One of the most important forms of cell death
is apoptosis. Collections of events force abnormal cells to fall on
their swords in service to the organism as a whole. Recognizing that
cancer hijacks normal physiology in service of its own needs, however detrimental to the patient, grants us a new perspective on this
and other illnesses.

In biology and in scientific discovery, indeed in virtually all
aspects of life, there are different mind-sets. As mentioned in chapter 22, we use the term "splitters" to describe those who dissect
every phenomenon down to its rudiments and focus on minute distinctions, and the term "lumpers" to describe those who coalesce
phenomena into larger groupings, seeking commonalities and sim-
ilarities. In medicine there is a joke that describes different medical
disciplines. On the one hand are the generalists (general practitioners) who come to know less and less about more and more until they
know nothing about everything. On the other hand are the specialists who know more and more about less and less until they know
everything about nothing.

We have come to admire, sponsor, and support the specialists.
These rarified academics spend entire careers defining SNP (single-
nucleotide polymorphism) or a transition from arginine to methio-
nine (two amino acids in proteins) within the ATP binding site of an
enzyme as their *raison d'état*. They get awards and receive stipends

but never once connect the dots that bridge one important discovery to another. They are the quintessential modern-day investigators. I, for one, believe that we have overvalued the contributions of the specialists and pride myself among the ranks of the lumpers.

Meaningful discoveries come from people who connect dots. Those rare, eclectic few who see patterns where others see blurs.We are chastised for being "unfocused." It's hard to get grants to study big ideas when little ideas are so much more easily quantified by grant-reviewing committees. Yet, it is big thinkers who cut across disciplines who make the discoveries that change the course of human history. Linus Pauling received two Nobel Prizes: the Peace Prize in 1962 and the Nobel Prize in Chemistry in 1954. Bruce Ames has influenced our understanding of human metabolism and free radical chemistry, and also invented the standard test used to measure whether common chemicals and medicines are likely to cause mutations and, thereby, cancer. This method, used around the world, bears his name—the Ames test.

Human biology is a very "lumpy" pursuit. In tissue cultures, cells clump together. Even individual cells lump functions together. In the study of protein chemistry, one will occasionally come across a truly miraculous finding that makes this fact abundantly clear. For example, the chemotherapy drug capecitabine is an oral formulation of the widely used drug 5-FU. Starting off as a prodrug (precursor) tablet, it goes through three separate enzymatic conversions within the body, winding up at the level of the cancer cell as 5-FU. The last enzyme in this cascade is thymidine phosphorylase. What I find extraordinary is the fact that thymidine phosphorylase is exactly the same protein as the molecule endothelial growth factor, a substance that promotes blood vessel formation in tumors. The exact same molecule. A drug-metabolizing enzyme is a blood vessel growth factor? It seems far-fetched. Ironically, this growth factor that cancer cells use to survive when stressed is the very enzyme that oncologists use to deliver cancer-killing 5-FU to the cell. It's like cleaning your dishes with your table scraps, but it works.

THE APOPTOSIS CONNECTION

Early in gestation and during the first years of life, the human body conditions its immune system. Lymphocytes are educated. Circulating through the thymus, cells are exposed to antigens. Glucocorticoids and the cytokine interleukin 3—when present at exactly the same instant within the cell—select these memory lymphocytes for cell survival. However, if this dual exposure does not occur with simultaneous precision, those lymphocytes suffer an apoptotic death. The death sentence is handed down to any errant immune cell that confuses friend with foe. The foes, in this case, are foreign proteins, bacteria, and viruses that are the targets of immune surveillance. But woe be the cell that stages an assault on those proteins that make you *you*. These self-antigens must be carefully preserved and can never be confused with the enemy. After all, you do not want to be at war with your own immune system.

Despite these safeguards, an occasional lymphocyte escapes the selection process and slowly amplifies. Years later (often decades), these mutinous lymphocytes mount an insurrection that we recognize as systemic lupus erythematosus (SLE), rheumatoid arthritis (RA), Hashimoto's disease, or any one of a number of other autoimmune disorders. These disease states reflect once again a dysregulation of cell death and failure of apoptosis.

For the latter part of the twentieth century, the leading cause of death in the United States was cardiovascular disease. Cardiologists were trained to study lipid levels, monitor lipoproteins, angiographically examine blood flow through arteries—all the while attempting to prevent atherosclerotic disease. Atherosclerosis occurs when immune cells, known as macrophages, become engorged with fat molecules, accumulate calcium, and ultimately attract platelets that block blood flow, leading to heart attacks and strokes.

But what drives the cells that line the blood vessels (known as endothelial cells) to proliferate? We now recognize that the inner lining of the blood vessels (known as the intimal layer) are subject to the same life-death cycles as all other tissues in the body. When the normal program of cell death fails, these tiny cells accumulate one upon another ultimately blocking the very blood flow they were designed to promote. Thus, atherosclerosis reflects the same changes in apoptotic signals within cells that we associate with cancer. Not surprisingly, cancer chemotherapeutic agents—like Taxol—are now routinely found in the drug-eluting stents used to treat coronary artery disease, while cholesterol-lowering drugs like Lipitor (and other statins), as well as therapies for diabetes like metformin, are showing up in protocols for the treatment and prevention of cancer. Once again we see commonality of human maladies driven by the process of programmed cell death.

Neurological diseases range from congenital and traumatic to a host of metabolic abnormalities. Among the most devastating of these disorders is Lou Gehrig's disease, or amyotrophic lateral sclerosis (ALS). This unrelenting scourge deprives people in the prime of their lives of the use of their muscles. It begins with rippling movements and progresses to complete loss of function (known as flaccidity). We now know that this disease is associated with oxygen free-radical activity within the neuron associated with the deficiency of an enzyme known as superoxide dismutase (SOD). SOD is essential for life in an oxygen-rich environment such as ours. The incapacity of neural cells to scavenge these free-radical super oxides triggers the process of programmed cell death and the slow loss of neurological function. Similar events are known to occur in the basal ganglia of the brain, resulting in Parkinson's disease. Indeed, many neurological disorders reflect hyperactive programmed cell death within the brain, spinal cord, and nerves. These are examples of common human diseases driven by too much programmed cell death.

THE ANSWERS ARE IN OUR METABOLISM

In 1982, a strange disease entity arose in certain New York and San Francisco communities. The illness seemed to afflict young men and was characterized by bizarre opportunistic infections, diminished white blood counts, weight loss, diarrhea, dementia, and unusual malignancies like Kaposi's sarcoma and B-cell non-Hodgkin lymphoma—all culminating in death within a year of diagnosis. This was AIDS (acquired immunodeficiency syndrome). What caused it, how to treat it, and how it was spread all remained a mystery. And then, two investigators—one in the United States and one in France—identified a transmissible, infectious agent, the human immunodeficiency virus (HIV). With that discovery, we recognized a novel virus of the RNA-type. Years later, antiretroviral drugs were developed and the disease came under better control.

AIDS, we came to realize, occurred when the HIV virus afflicted one subset of lymphocytes known as CD4-positive cells. These so-called "helper" lymphocytes were responsible for amplifying immune response to infectious agents. Lymphocyte proliferation and response to antigens is a complicated collection of signaling events, protein synthesis, and increased metabolic activity. HIV-infected lymphocytes, when called upon to respond, instead died. These cells, it seemed, committed suicide when they were called upon to defend the body as a whole. By mechanisms not quite fully understood, an increase of free radical activity within these cells triggered programmed cell death and the resultant immune dysregulation.

Recognizing the principal role of altered, free-radical chemistry within these cells, my colleague Dr. Sheldon Hendler suggested a solution. Would it be possible, he reasoned, to dampen the storm of oxygen radicals released at the time of immune stimulation? Could we protect these delicate cells and maintain immune function? He suggested that free-radical scavengers might do the job, but vitamin C, selenium, and most of the usual suspects, had provided little benefit for the afflicted patients. He needed something that would get into the cells and deliver the needed protection but carry little toxicity. To accomplish the goal, he identified a drug previously used in the management of hypercholesterolemia. Together with Robert Sanchez, PhD, they dissolved this chemical in a mid-chain fatty acid formulation and Panavir R was born.

Dr. Hendler and I collaborated on a Phase I clinical trial. This novel concept worked beautifully and provided evidence of a meaningful improvement in HIV-positive patients' lymphocyte counts and viral loads. Some of the patients treated with this novel approach are alive today twenty years later. Despite our success, the FDA was not interested. It seems that protease inhibitors were in style that year and our therapeutic intervention, however effective, was cut from a different cloth. This nontoxic drug failed to garner the attention and support it needed to sponsor further trials, and it died on the vine. Nonetheless, as a proof of concept, this experience was a beautiful success. By modulating free radical oxygen activity within the intracellular environment, we had proven that one could stanch oxygen-triggered cell death. This remains a key component of my thinking and the thinking of other researchers as we move to the era of metabolomic medicine.

As a resident of Southern California, I reside in a part of the country that can best be described as a desert by the sea. The arid landscape of this region reveals plush greenery limited exclusively to those areas where irrigation is provided. Just inches from the hydraulic spout, the scorched earth resembles a Martian landscape centuries removed from its last contact with water.

Despite this depravation, several times a year tropical Pacific storms blow eastward bringing with them torrential downfalls, sometimes at the rate of several inches per hour. Suddenly, the Department of Public Works is called upon to control flash floods in this erstwhile barren clime.

To most, floods and droughts are diametric opposites, characterized by too much and too little water respectively. Similarly, to the scientific "splitter," cancer and AIDS are opposites, characterized by too little or too much cell death. But, to the scientific "lumper," these seemingly disparate phenomena are nothing more than opposite ends of the same spectrum.

Civil engineers, recognizing the need for more intelligent resource management, constructed reservoirs, aqueducts, and culverts to retain water in times of drought and channel its flow in times of flood. The analogy with human disease states is an apt one, for physicians of the future will learn to regulate the ebb and flow of life forces to balance the excesses, not unlike their engineering brethren.

For the past century, physicists have pursued a unified field theory to connect quantum mechanics to Newtonian physics. Medical scientists must redouble their efforts to identify commonalities that connect disease entities if they are ultimately to develop more effective treatments.

The concept of programmed cell death, for me, opened a window onto human tumor biology that extended well beyond cancer to virtually all other human diseases. It provided an opportunity to reexamine cancer biology with regard to DNA, RNA, and genomics in the context of bioenergetics and physiology. Using membrane integrity and cellular metabolism as my probes, I came to realize based on my observations that the driving force of cancer was energy. I became increasingly convinced that cancer was, indeed, a disease of cellular energy, not informatics.

My interest in chemistry and love of biochemistry, and my many hours of discussion with Dr. Hendler and others, made it increasingly clear that cancer developed as a perturbation in bioenergetics. The cure for cancer will be had when we depart from our fixation on cellular informatics and the nucleus, and return to the study of energy production and its principal organelle—the mitochondrion.

As the scales fall away from our eyes, we will see that it is not just cancer, but all disease, that reflects changes in metabolism. In this way, cancer will prove to be a portal that guides us to discoveries that address all human diseases.

APPENDICES

Cancer Research Explained

There are many reasons why medical oncologists may not use laboratory-directed approaches for the treatment of their patients. The arguments against these approaches tend to differ by practice type. Academic physicians have chosen a career within the ivory tower setting of university medical centers. These physicians have been trained to believe that enrolling as many patients as possible into clinical trials will help them to achieve the highest level of accomplishment in the field.

These clinical trials, also known as protocols, are broken down into three distinct categories.

The first, known as Phase I trials, examine the tolerability of drugs in humans. As these drugs move into the clinic directly from pre-clinical and animal models, no one knows whether they can safely be given to humans. Thus, Phase I trials are designed to determine proper dosages and to examine the capacity of patients to tolerate the drug but have little (if any) focus on therapeutic benefit. The investigators engaged in Phase I trials are a sturdy breed, for they enter into an absolute unknown with every new drug. They confront the sickest of all patients, as it is only those most desperate patients who will agree to clinical trials without the expectation of response. These investigators are found at major universities because only those institutions have the supporting infrastructure to conduct the studies required by the FDA. These Phase I investigators serve a vital function, one that I cannot duplicate or improve upon in the laboratory. As a regular attendee at the National Cancer Institute Phase I meetings for many years, I was always impressed by the scientific acumen and dedication of these physicians. I, for one, indeed all medical oncologists and cancer patients, owe them a debt of gratitude for their hard work and the high-quality data that they generate.

The second tier of cancer drug development falls upon the Phase II trial physicians. Gleaning crucial information from their Phase I colleagues about dose and schedule, these physicians take the drugs that they know they can give and try to determine whom to give them to. While doses and schedules may differ among Phase II trials of the same drug, the principal intent is to achieve a 20 percent objective response rate (that is, 20 out of every 100 patients treated show clinical improvement). The clinical trials themselves are designed to quickly throw out "bad" drugs and promote "good" drugs. These protocols seek benefit wherever it exists so that they can conclude the trial as quickly as possible and move on to the next candidate drug.

Phase II trials are also largely conducted at academic centers but have, over recent years, extended into the clinical community through cooperative groups and large practice organizations. They are lucrative, popular, and largely unsuccessful. A distinct minority of new drugs demonstrate effectiveness. Indeed, according to one study published in the *New England Journal of Medicine* (Roberts 2003) only 8 percent of drugs that complete Phase I go on to achieve adequate therapeutic benefit and earn FDA approval.

It is this area of clinical investigation that could most benefit from the intelligent application of laboratory-based therapeutics. Yet, it is this moderately large group of academic physicians who are the most entrenched in their refusal to use our approach. The Phase II physicians blindly administer drugs under protocols developed and distributed by pharmaceutical companies. These physicians, whether academic or university affiliates, resist change and continue the random administration of chemotherapeutics—however little benefit it may provide their patients. As Janet Woodcock from the FDA has described it, "Our understanding of biomedical science has far exceeded our capacity to test drugs." She has defined the failure to connect gee-whiz scientists with successful clinical outcomes as the need for a "critical path from bench to bedside." (American Associaton for Cancer Research, Special Symposium on Drug Development, Annual Meeting, June 2006) I believe that our laboratory platform is just that critical path.

The final group of physicians are those engaged in Phase III trials. Once we know that a drug can be given (Phase I) and to whom we should give it (Phase II), we need to know whether the new drug is better than the existing drugs. This duty falls to the Phase III trialists. Under the auspices of large cooperative groups with names like National Surgical Adjuvant Breast and Bowel Project (NSABP), a patchwork of hospitals and doctors all over the U.S. participate in large, multi-institutional studies. These trials are little more than numbers games. Bristol-Myers Squibb wants to prove that ixabepilone is as good as or better than paclitaxel. Or Eli Lilly and Company wants to prove that carboplatin plus gemcitabine is as good as carboplatin plus paclitaxel. These are the studies that most second- and third-tier medical institutions promote in their brochures as "cancer research."

Despite the fanfare, only one in seven clinical trials of this type reveal the superiority of the new drug "A" over the older drug "B" (Soares 2006). More disturbing is the fact that only one out of fourteen of these trials improves the survival of the patients so treated by 50 percent or more; usually by days, sometimes weeks; rarely months and never years. (Djulbegovic 2006).

With the exception of the Phase I trials, the purpose of which is to determine whether drugs can be given and how to give them, the rest of the clinical trial process is in desperate need of an overhaul. It has become a bloated bureaucracy that provides sponsorship and support, opportunity and advance, academic and financial enrichment, and benefits everyone involved except the patient.

Cancer patients aren't cannon fodder (cannon fodder is an informal, derogatory term for military personnel who are regarded or treated as expendable in the face of enemy fire). It is not their duty to be martyred at the altar of drug development. As medical oncologists, we should do everything within our power to make sure that no patient receives a drug unless we feel confident that it has a good chance of working.

While I cannot guarantee an outcome based upon my work, I can, on average, double the likelihood of a clinical response when a drug appears active in the test tube. We have shown this in peer review published literature for more than two decades. I have personally contributed statistically significant data in breast, ovarian, and lung cancers, and in childhood leukemia; my colleagues and associates have done the same in small cell lung cancer, adult leukemia, and, somewhat surprisingly, malignant melanoma. The data is available and irrefutable. What is disturbing is that it isn't being used effectively.

What to Expect When You're Expecting a Conversation with Your Oncologist

Part of the reason why I have written this book is to empower patients to make smart clinical decisions and take charge of their own cancer. As I say to every one of my patients, "No one is more interested in saving your life than you."

A patient interested in using laboratory-directed therapy typically confronts a laundry list of reasons why it shouldn't be used. For the benefit of the reader, I provide an outline of the typical arguments that a patient may encounter.

Physician: This type of testing has been tried before and it was proven not to work.

Response: In the past, drug sensitivity testing was conducted in artificial models that grew cancer cells. After stimulating the cells to grow, these tests measured the capacity of chemotherapy drugs to stop cells from growing. It didn't work, we agree. The reasons why it didn't work are a large part of this book. Suffice it to say that in the modern era, our understanding of programmed cell death has led us to recognize that cancer cells don't grow too much, they die too little. Measuring cancer growth in test tubes is not only misguided, it's irrelevant. These tests did not work, could not work, and failed for reasons that are now abundantly obvious. We do not grow cells.

Physician: What works in the test tube won't work in the patient.

Response: It is not the intent of laboratory tests to re-create the human body in a test tube. Obviously, there is no immune system, kidney, heart, or brain in a 1cc tube. But cancer tests are designed to measure the most fundamental aspect of drug response—the ability of cells to die following exposure to drugs.

The way a drug is given, the role of the immune system, and drug metabolism all contribute to the effectiveness of a treatment. But if the therapy, under optimal conditions, cannot kill the cancer cells, then the patient won't respond.

These laboratory models have been calibrated to provide information that reflects human response. The drug concentrations and conditions of exposure are not intended to mimic the body. Instead, under controlled and highly reproducible conditions, the drug exposure in the test tube has been shown to predict response in the patient.

The disinterested observer might inquire, "Why don't you add bleach to the test tube?" My response would be that bleach, of course, kills cancer cells. In fact, along the same lines, it is actually very easy to cure cancer. The problem is that no patients would survive the treatments. Obviously, cancer therapies are administered within the confines of tolerable doses. Bleach, like cyanide or arsenic or, for that matter, boiling water, will kill every cancer cell. The role of the laboratory test, therefore, is to measure the activity of a drug with a direct connection to patient outcomes. The raw data that comes from the laboratory is analyzed against hundreds of thousands of data points, enabling us to compare that degree of drug effect with hundreds or thousands of prior patients. Although it is not perfect, a drug selected in the laboratory is twice as likely to work as one randomly selected by your physician.

Physician: The tests are good at telling you what won't work, but can't tell you what will.

Response: This is another example of old thinking clouding contemporary discussion. What these physicians are referring to is the growth-based assay model (see previous). These older tests artificially stimulated cancer cells to reproduce. Only then were the cells exposed to drugs. It is not surprising in retrospect that these growing cells had a strong tendency to stop growing when they were poisoned. After all, if someone plucked you out of your home, dropped you naked into a vat of warm broth, and suggested you start a family, you might also decline. When these cancer cells didn't choose to grow, the investigators interpreted this to mean that the drugs were active. This is the reason that these tests so frequently identified sensitivity. There was virtually no discriminating capacity, except for one circumstance—when cancer cells plucked from their warm environment, dumped into broth, and exposed to toxic substances (chemotherapies) nonetheless decided to raise a family. These comparatively rare but truly drug-resistant cancer cells proved themselves capable of growing under the most extreme conditions. For that reason, truly drug-resistant populations could be identified as bad candidates for therapy even using the worst of tests.

While it is true that a very small percentage of cancers could be identified in this manner (the so-called extreme drug-resistant group) the information was just this side of useless. After all, most cancer patients don't respond very well to chemotherapy and we certainly don't need help finding bad drugs. There are already plenty of those around. What patients need is help finding drugs that work. It turns out that that information can best be obtained by measuring cell death in nongrowing cells with their guard up and defenses ready.

You don't go to a restaurant to find out what they aren't serving. You don't go to an airport to find out where they aren't flying. And you don't go to your oncologist to find out what treatment not to take. Laboratory assays that measure growth and proliferation can only tell you what not to get. That is why I departed from that technology two decades ago to use newer, more accurate techniques and will never go back.

Physician: You'll lose valuable time awaiting the results of the test.

Response: Patients who are newly diagnosed with cancer must undergo a series of diagnostic tests and interventions. These usually include blood tests, tumor markers, complete staging, and special studies conducted on their tumor biopsies. All of these tests usually require one to two weeks before a patient can begin treatment. Ex-vivo analyses are short-term tissue culture techniques that can be completed within one week.

Contrary to older methodologies based upon cell proliferation (growth), cell death assays require only several days for completion. While the older techniques could require weeks, a month, or more to provide results, programmed cell death measurements are available within a week. This turnaround time ensures that the recommendations will be available as soon as the patient is ready for treatment. As we say to our patients, "It is better to wait one week to receive the right treatment than to receive the wrong treatment today."

Physician: The best treatment for you is the standard of care for your disease.

Response: The operative term here is "standard." Today, medical oncologists are increasingly encouraged to adhere to the standards defined in the National Comprehensive Cancer Network (NCCN) guidelines. These treatment protocols provide up-to-date recommendations for treatments by diagnosis. One might define this as the "average patient, average outcome" approach. Average outcomes are what these guidelines are designed to provide and they're exactly what you get.

Our mission is to disrupt this tidy model through the use of objective data to select active drugs. As there are no truly average patients, there are no truly average outcomes. While the NCCN guidelines represent the "one size fits all" approach, we see their results as "one size fits none." For example, the well-established response rate in advanced non-small cell lung cancer of 31 percent does not reflect a 31 percent shrinkage in everyone's tumor. Instead, 31 out of every 100 patients enjoy some benefit, while the remaining 69 suffer only toxicity.

The intent of laboratory analysis is to divide these "average patients" into two groups: those more and those less likely to respond. As we have shown repeatedly, assay-directed therapies will approximately double the likelihood of a clinical response in assay-positive patients.

No test is perfect. No response is guaranteed. But given the wealth of data supporting these approaches, what patient confronting a life or death situation wouldn't want to double their odds of response to treatment?

Physician: The tests are costly and not reimbursed by insurance.

Response: Cancer therapy is expensive. The average patient receives treatments that cost thousands of dollars per dose with additional tens of thousands of dollars in diagnostic, therapeutic, and supportive measures. An analysis that examined the cost of treatment for patients with advanced colon cancer found that as these costs continue to skyrocket, they could soon surpass society's capacity to sponsor these therapies (Ferro 2008). Proposed political solutions to address these spiraling costs include limited access (restriction to on-label use, third-party payer policy, etc.) or outright rationed care.

All of these draconian measures reflect the broad-brush approval process that grants access to drugs in the first place. Patients with a given diagnosis, stage, and treatment history have access to a given therapy, while those one stage above or below are not allowed to receive the benefit. It's arbitrary, it's unscientific, and it isn't working.

To counter this approach, we offer rational drug selection. Patients receive treatments found effective for their individual disease. Patients found drug-resistant receive other treatments or are referred to experimental therapies early enough in their illnesses to tolerate investigational drugs. The cost of laboratory analyses pale in comparison to the mounting costs of ineffective therapy, particularly when one factors in the lost time, increased toxicities, and opportunity costs associated with the wrong drugs.

A Practical Guide for the Use of Chemosensitivity Testing

Despite protestations to the contrary, the oncologic community must admit that there is no *right* treatment for any cancer. With the exception of gestational choriocarcinoma, a rare form of gynecologic malignancy for which methotrexate plus actinomycin D is uniformly effective, all other cancer patients have choices. Cancer medicine, it seems, is subject to the same types of trends that drive women's fashion. Like fitted suits or short skirts, doxorubicin for breast cancer is in and then it's out—so yesterday. But it will be back again.

All the while, patients suffer through dose intensity, dose density, bone marrow transplantation, and targeted therapies only to find out that the conceptual underpinnings that led their doctor to treat them accordingly were wrong and everyone's going back to the drawing board. This happens because there are no absolutes in drug selection. There is only opinion, and opinions vary.

While the cut of my trousers or width of my tie is a matter of personal preference, the outcome of my patients is demonstrably more than a fashion. Good taste is always in style and good therapy always works. Patients deserve good therapy.

To remove the subjectivity of drug selection, we have introduced the objective data of drug-response profiling. While the average patient with lung cancer in the United States in 2012 might be a

candidate for carboplatin plus pemetrexed with or without bevacizumab, I absolutely guarantee that many of them would do better with something else. The same is true for patients with ovarian
cancer who received carboplatin plus paclitaxel or breast cancer
patients who receive cyclophosphamide plus docetaxel. Into this
opinion-driven mix we throw rational therapeutics.

So let's examine, by disease, how a laboratory analysis might
influence the drug selection for a given patient.

COLON CANCER

We'll start with colon cancer. Here is a disease that languished in
obscurity for forty years. Following the development of 5-FU, every
patient with colon cancer received this drug. Then, in the 1980s, the
addition of leucovorin, a reduced form of B vitamin, increased the
response rate and provided a new standard of care. From the rather
dismal 12 to 14 percent response rates observed for two decades, 20
percent of patients who received 5-FU plus leucovorin were now
responding. In the 1990s, irinotecan—a modification of an old drug
known as camptothecin, resurrected by Japanese investigators—
arrived on the scene and patients who had failed 5-FU plus leucovorin had a new option. Then came oxaliplatin, followed by
cetuximab and bevacizumab. Then French investigators put 5-FU
together with oxaliplatin and leucovorin and the FOLFOX regimen
was born.

Today, a patient with advanced colon cancer might receive:

- FOLFOX (5-FU plus leucovorin plus oxaliplatin)

- FOLFIRI (5-FU plus irinotecan)

- 5-FU/leucovorin

- IROX (irinotecan plus oxaliplatin)

- FOLFOX plus bevacizumab

- FOLFOX plus cetuximab

- FOLFIRI plus bevacizumab

- FOLFIRI plus cetuximab

- Irinotecan plus bevacizumab plus cetuximab

As you can see, there is no right treatment for this diagnosis.

BREAST CANCER

The earliest evidence of activity for breast cancer patients came in the 1950s when single agent alkylators were administered. Italian investigators then combined cyclophosphamide with methotrexate with 5-FU (CMF) providing the first truly effective combination for this disease. To this was added Adriamycin and later the taxanes and vinorelbine. With the discovery of the HER-2 oncogene, trastuzumab entered clinical therapy. And finally, late to the game, came the platins (both carboplatin and cisplatin) joined by gemcitabine, capecitabine, and a host of combinations.

Today, a newly diagnosed breast cancer patient might receive:

- CA (cyclophosphamide plus Adriamycin)

- CAF (cyclophosphamide plus Adriamycin plus 5-FU)

- CMF (cyclophosphamide plus methotrexate plus 5-FU)

- Cyclophosphamide plus docetaxel

- CA followed by docetaxel

- CA followed by Taxol

- Docetaxel plus capecitabine

- Docetaxel plus gemcitabine

- Paclitaxel plus gemcitabine

- Single agent capecitabine

- Vinorelbine plus capecitabine

- Carboplatin plus Taxol

- Carboplatin plus docetaxel

- Carboplatin plus docetaxel plus trastuzumab

- Liposomal doxorubicin

- Lapatinib

OVARIAN CANCER

Although this may be the single most chemoresponsive cancer that medical oncologists regularly treat, the cure rates for this disease have changed little in several decades. Might this reflect our insistence that every patient with this diagnosis receive carboplatin plus paclitaxel?

Despite the inability of the cooperative group system to distinguish carboplatin plus paclitaxel from other combinations in the now famous GOG-182 clinical trial that accrued 4,312 patients to five different treatment arms—to find no difference among the arms (Bookman 2009)—there is every reason to believe that selecting amongst those treatment options might have provided a different outcome.

For first-line therapy, the options, well established for their equivalence, include:

- Carboplatin plus paclitaxel

- Carboplatin plus docetaxel

- Carboplatin plus liposomal doxorubicin

- Carboplatin plus gemcitabine

- Single agent carboplatin

- Cyclophosphamide plus doxorubicin plus cisplatin (CAP)

Despite there being no data to establish the superiority of any of the above-listed regimens over another, every patient in the United States diagnosed with advanced ovarian cancer will receive carboplatin plus paclitaxel.

While the first-line options may seem confusing, it's all downhill from there when the disease recurs. A nonexhaustive list of treatment options for recurrent disease is provided below:

- Liposomal doxorubicin

- Topotecan

- Carboplatin plus paclitaxel

- Carboplatin plus docetaxel

- Carboplatin plus liposomal doxorubicin

- Carboplatin plus gemcitabine

- Single agent carboplatin

- Paclitaxel

- Docetaxel

- Gemcitabine

- Vinorelbine

- Capecitabine

- Melphalan

- FOLFOX

- Liposomal doxorubicin plus gemcitabine

- Cyclophosphamide plus topotecan

And the list goes on.

LUNG CANCER

Lung cancer splits into two principal subcategories: small cell lung cancer and non-small cell lung cancer.

For small cell lung cancer, drugs with measurable activity include:

- Cyclophosphamide

- Ifosfamide

- Doxorubicin

- Irinotecan

- Topotecan

- Etoposide

- Carboplatin

- Cisplatin

As well as the widely used combinations of:

- Cisplatin plus etoposide

- Cisplatin plus irinotecan

- Carboplatin plus etoposide

- Carboplatin plus irinotecan

With non-small cell lung cancer, the options only expand. We'll focus primarily upon combinations, as they are the most widely used:

- Cisplatin plus paclitaxel

- Carboplatin plus paclitaxel

- Cisplatin plus vinorelbine

- Carboplatin plus vinorelbine
- Cisplatin plus gemcitabine
- Carboplatin plus gemcitabine
- Cisplatin plus docetaxel
- Carboplatin plus docetaxel
- Cisplatin plus pemetrexed
- Carboplatin plus pemetrexed
- Cisplatin plus irinotecan
- Carboplatin plus irinotecan
- Cisplatin plus etoposide
- Carboplatin plus etoposide
- Docetaxel plus gemcitabine

In addition, single agents might be considered, including:

- Docetaxel
- Paclitaxel
- Pemetrexed
- Vinorelbine
- Gemcitabine
- Irinotecan
- Erlotinib
- Crizotinib

OTHER CANCERS

While we could carry this line of discussion on through every disease from mesothelioma to malignant melanoma, the point is: cancer patients have options. Narrowing these options down to those most likely to work is what Rational Therapeutics does. We and a small coterie of dedicated clinical investigators have continued to apply these life-saving methodologies in the service of their patients. Based upon the well-established performance characteristics—known as sensitivity and specificity—these tests can, on average, double the likelihood of a good outcome for any given patient.

SENSITIVITY AND SPECIFICITY DEFINED

Sensitivity describes the ability of a test to find what it's looking for. Like radar detecting enemy aircraft or a chest x-ray diagnosing tuberculosis, sensitive tests identify all potential candidates. The problem with an overly sensitive test is just that. They identify *all* potential candidates. A very sensitive radar screen will detect every flying object, from an enemy bomber to a mosquito. Bringing this back to cancer therapy testing—a very sensitive drug evaluation test would suggest that every patient tested might benefit from the drug in question. As in the military context, where distinguishing bombers from mosquitos has profound implications, suggesting that everyone might respond to a drug has no discriminating ability and, therefore, no utility.

The flip side of the coin is specificity. This is defined as the capacity of a test to rule out the likelihood of a given finding. Let's use the radar analogy to explore the concept. A highly specific radar technology would ratchet up the gain to the point where only the largest of large crafts would be detected, ultimately missing everything but the Goodyear Blimp. While one would reliably know that danger existed when the screen detected an entity with the dimensions of a zeppelin, this would miss a large percentage of enemy aircraft and, again, fail to provide help to those entrusted to protect their nation. Returning to the cancer therapy environment, an overly specific test would exclude all but the most sensitive patients and, again, fail to provide utility.

In the field of medicine, all tests must be adjusted to balance sensitivity (finding it when it is there) against specificity (eliminating it when it's not). Over the years, we have calibrated our tests to provide sensitivities and specificities in the range of 80 to 90 percent. We readily accept some errors at either extreme so that the majority of patients can be accurately characterized. Few patients realize that all medical tests are similarly calibrated. For example, a widely used test for blood chemistry is known as a comprehensive metabolic profile (CMP). This collection of twenty separate blood tests, run simultaneously, is calibrated to 95 percent accuracy. Put slightly differently, 5 percent of the time, the test is wrong. In real terms, this means that one out of every twenty CMP values is likely to be incorrect. That elevated potassium or mildly low immunoglobulin level may be an error, not a cause for alarm.

While we are accustomed to these error bars on many medical tests, the medical oncology community has tended to hold in vitro chemosensitivity testing to a higher standard. That is, every patient found sensitive must respond and every patient found resistant cannot. This patently ridiculous standard is the reason many clinicians eschew these useful tests. "I tried it once and the patient didn't respond to the recommended drug," is what a patient might hear. Were that same physician to say, "I did an x-ray but it didn't diagnose the lung cancer, so I'll never do an x-ray again," the average patient would recognize the fallacy of this reasoning. X-rays miss cancers. Blood tests make errors. And cancer chemosensitivity tests double response rates, but they don't provide a perfect solution to every cancer patient's problems.

APPENDIX D

Assay Criteria

Approximately 1.4 million Americans are diagnosed with cancer each year. Of those, almost half will be treated with some form of chemotherapy or molecularly targeted agent. With so many drug choices for each cancer type, it makes sense for you to have the best information possible for treating your disease.

STEP 1—THE QUALIFICATIONS

We can test patients who are newly diagnosed, as well as those who have had a recurrence or whose cancer has spread. To ensure the accuracy of our results, patients must be off active chemotherapy or radiation at the time the sample is collected. Generally, a two- to four-week break between treatment and biopsy is recommended.

STEP 2—OBTAINING A SAMPLE

At Rational Therapeutics, we do not grow or subculture cells in the laboratory. This guarantees the most accurate results for your assay. While some laboratories amplify or propagate biopsy specimens, this changes the cancer cells' behavior and selects out subpopulations that may not be reflective of your own cancer biology. Since we do not grow (expand) your cells, we need to obtain a large enough sample at the beginning to test all the drugs of interest. A needle biopsy is not enough.

Quantity of specimen required:

- Solid tumor—a minimum of one gram (one cubic centimeter) of viable malignant tissue.

- Blood (leukemia)—a minimum of ten milliliters (about two tubes).

- Bone marrow (leukemia and myeloma)—one to three milliliters of first pull or a separate aspirate into a pre-heparinized syringe.

- Malignant effusions (pleural or ascites fluids)—500 to 1,000 milliliters of fluid with a tumor cell percentage greater than 30 and the ratio of tumor to reactive mesothelial cells should be greater than 2 to 1. Twenty thousand units of heparin should be added to each liter bottle.

STEP 3—SENDING YOUR SAMPLE TO RATIONAL THERAPEUTICS

If a surgical procedure is scheduled, you can call us for a kit and instructions for your surgeon on how to properly send the sample. We need to receive the sample within twenty-four hours—while cells are still living—to perform your assay.

Between 85 and 95 percent of specimens received in our laboratory provide viable cells. On rare occasions, cells die en route to our laboratory. There are also times when a biopsy specimen that appeared malignant to the surgeon may not contain any cancer cells, or too few to test adequately.

If you plan to have your surgeon send a sample to our lab, please follow these instructions for packaging and shipping:

Solids and hematologic tumors:

1. Write the patient name, date, time, and specimen site on transport tube label.

2. Seal transport tube tightly.

3. Place specimen and Cold-Pak in transport box.

4. Enclose completed Requisition and Patient Information (face sheet or admitting record) and specimen transport box into FedEx "Diagnostic Specimen Envelope" and seal. Samples must be shipped FedEx Priority Overnight.

Fluid specimens:

1. Place fluid container inside the FedEx "Diagnostic Specimen Envelope" and seal.

2. Place specimen and completed Requisition and Patient Information (face sheet or admitting record) into transport box. Samples must be shipped FedEx Priority Overnight.

STEP 4—THE ASSAY

Once at Rational Therapeutics, your sample will be exposed to different drugs and combinations. Based on the quantity and quality of the sample, our laboratory will generally analyze your tumor's response against eight to sixteen drugs and combinations to identify which treatments will work best to cause your cancer to die. Results typically take seven to ten days from the time the sample is received at the laboratory.

STEP 5—THE RESULTS

Once your laboratory results have been analyzed, a detailed report

or "functional profile" is created. We send treatment recommendations directly to your oncologist. From there, you can work directly
with your physician to determine a treatment regimen that will
work for you.

Physician/Patient Advocate Resources

Ferre Akbarpour, MD, ABHM, ABAA
Hope Through Integrative Medicine for All Cancer Patients
Orange County Immune Institute
18800 Delaware Street
Huntington Beach, CA 92648
714-842-1777
www.drferre.com

Dr. Ferre applies scientifically validated alternative and complementary medicine approaches for chronic diseases that have been poorly addressed by traditional medical methods. In a caring, relaxed, and friendly environment, she provides stress and nutritional management, avoidance of toxicity, and the utilization of natural supplements for boosting or modeling the body's immune system.

Keith Block, MD
The Block Center
5230 Old Orchard Road
Skokie, IL 60077
877-41-BLOCK (412-5625)
847-492-3040
www.blockmd.com

In 1980, Keith Block, MD, and Penny Block, PhD, founded the Block Center for Integrative Cancer Treatment, the first center of its kind in the United States. From the inception, their mission has been to provide the kind of care they would each hope to receive, should they ever be faced with a diagnosis of cancer. The Block Center's services and treatment regimens—aimed at restoring biological integrity and laying the foundation essential to an enduring recovery—include: advanced laboratory and molecular testing; personalized nutrition and nutraceutical counseling; supportive mind-body training; prescriptive exercise instruction, innovative chemotherapy administration, including chronomodulated and metronomic infusion; targeted molecular treatments; off-label and experimental therapies and immunotherapies. In addition, the clinic provides training in therapeutic cooking, yoga, Qigong, massage, and group counseling in *Life Over Cancer* strategies.

The Center's staff includes board-certified oncologists and internists, physician assistants, oncology nurses, mind-spirit clinicians, psychologists, registered dietitians, physical therapists, licensed massage therapists, instructors in Asian fitness systems, medical researchers, and other integrative care specialists.

D. Barry Boyd, MD
15 Valley Drive
Greenwich, CT 06831
203-869-2111

With twenty-three years experience as a board-certified medical oncologist/hematologist and a Master's degree in nutritional biochemistry, Dr. Boyd specializes in cancer treatment and recovery. He is a pioneer in the field of integrative cancer care with a targeted focus on nutritional support for cancer patients. Incorporating emergent evidence-based medical oncology with cancer-specific nutritional counseling, Dr. Boyd combines comprehensive support for the healing process.

Henry Dreher, MA
Cancer Guide Consultations
84 East 3rd Street, #2C
New York, NY 10003
347-344-7057

Henry Dreher, is the director of Cancer Guide Consultations in New York City. In his capacity as a "Cancer Guide," Mr. Dreher conducts research for patients with all types of cancer, providing expert consultation on the most effective cancer treatments available. In phone consultations and written communications, he educates patients on the most promising therapies; guides them through the process of testing of their own tumor tissue for the design of personalized drug therapies; refers them to leading experts in their cancers; and empowers them to develop their own "team" of oncologic experts. He also helps patients to integrate scientifically grounded complementary therapies (nutrition, natural compounds, mind-body medicine, fitness, etc.) with cutting-edge mainstream therapies. With more than twenty-five years experience as a researcher, educator, and patient advocate, Mr. Dreher brings a unique body of knowledge to his practice. Dreher has authored nine books on topics from cancer prevention to integrative medicine to mind-body healing. His most recent book is *Mind-Body Unity: A New Vision for Mind-Body Science and Medicine* (Johns Hopkins University Press, 2003).

Marcia K. Horn, CEO
International Cancer Advocacy Network (ICAN)
27 West Morten Avenue
Phoenix, AZ 85021-7246
(By appointment only)
www.askican.org
602-618-0183
ProgramServices@askican.org

The International Cancer Advocacy Network (ICAN), headquartered in Phoenix and founded in 1996, is a 501(c)(3) charitable organization providing Stage IV cancer patients in the United States and 48 other countries with cutting-edge, creative, and tenacious information services, empowerment tools, and advocacy through its Personalized Medicine Cancer Case Management Programs. ICAN has a global network of more than 700 volunteers in twelve time zones. The organization refers patients to leading oncologists, as well as to treatment modalities that may have been overlooked by the patient's medical oncology team, such as surgical oncology, radiation oncology, or interventional radiology. ICAN also assists patients and their oncologists with clinical trial research, compassionate use (Single Patient IND) submissions, functional profiling of their tumor through Rational Therapeutics' platform EVA-PCD, and molecular profiling options, thus providing the patient with direct navigation at every step of his/her battle in the effort to extend life with the highest achievable quality of life. Profiled in *Newsweek* and in *Pharmaceutical Executive*, ICAN works closely with drug discoverers and drug development teams, clinicians, and oncology research scientists within and outside of ICAN to provide a "Tumor Board" approach for the most complex cases. Through its Remission Coach health information technology initiatives, ICAN is working on a search engine for late-stage patients as well as web-based apps and mobile apps for the general public.

Thomas Lodi, MD
An Oasis of Healing
210 N. Center St., Suite #102
Mesa, AZ 85201
480-834-5414
www.anoasisofhealing.com

An Oasis of Healing integrates scientifically validated, state-of-the-art cancer therapies with the healing traditions that have withstood the test of time. This includes traditional therapies from around the world, as well as conventional allopathic medicine. The basis for integrating these traditional modalities, alternative therapies, and conventional cancer treatments is developed through a thorough and continual study of and a reverence for nature. Even people with the same type of cancers have unique requirements; therefore, everyone has a plan of care that is individualized. For this reason, the staff relies on Rational Therapeutics to provide a chemotherapeutic regimen specific to each patient's unique requirements.

Ralph Moss, PhD
Cancer Decisions
800-980-1234 or 814-238-4064
email anne@cancerdecisions.com
www.cancerdecisions.com

Cancer Decisions has many ways to help provide patients with up-to-date information on cancer treatments. Their website offers individual Moss Reports on specific types of cancers. Their monthly electronic newsletter, ADVANCES in Cancer Treatment, is written by Ralph W. Moss, PhD. Phone consultations are available to those who purchase a Moss Report on their type of cancer. Their professional associate program offers patients information on healthcare providers in their local area. They also offer many videos about their programs, products, and a video blog. The Cancer Decisions Newsletter archives contains ten years of weekly newsletters about news and the treament of cancer. Books and visualization audios are also available.

Mark Renneker, MD
University of California, San Francisco
415-681-5357

Dr. Renneker is a university-affiliated, board-certified family physician providing clinical advocacy help to patients and families dealing with complex and life-threatening illnesses, particularly cancer. San Francisco–based, the doctor performs most of his consultations by phone, with patients and family members around the country (and world). He practices what he calls "optimistic medicine," that no matter how desperate or hopeless a situation may appear, there are always new approaches to consider, and he is good at finding, evaluating, and helping implement such strategies, drawing from all fields of medicine: mainstream, experimental, and integrative. Taking such a "no stone unturned" approach when seeking to explore cutting edge therapies, he has often worked successfully with Dr. Nagourney. Payment is out of pocket, simply for his time, using a sliding scale.

Gwendolyn Stritter, MD
3130 Alpine Road #288
Portola Valley, CA 94028
650-851-0377

Dr. Gwendolyn Stritter is a double-board certified physician who, since the summer of 2000, has practiced clinical advocacy—a unique consulting practice for those seeking everything from personalized research to finding the right medical team. A pioneer in the clinical advocacy field, she co-wrote a chapter in the 2007 textbook *Patient Advocacy* (Jossey-Bass, publisher; J Earp, editor), detailing how such a practice helps patients and families facing complex, life-threatening illnesses. Her special interests include breast and gynecologic cancers.

Robert Zieve, MD
EuroMed Foundation
34975 North Valley Parkway
Bldg. 6, Suite 138
Phoenix, AZ 85086
602-404-0400
www.euro-med.us

Dr. Zieve is supervising physician at the EuroMed Foundation Integrative Cancer Clinic in Phoenix, Arizona, which specializes in treating cancer with insulin potentiation therapy (IPT). He integrates homeopathy, botanical medicine, neural therapy, nutrition, and intravenous therapies. He is certified in the use of IPT. Dr. Zieve is highly trained in applying botanical and nutritional/dietary regimens to patients with cancer, in ways that highly individualize care. Dr. Zieve has trained in integrative oncology with nationally recognized oncologists. He is medical director of the Healthy Medicine Academy, which conducts annual conferences in integrative cancer medicine (http://healthymedicineacademy.com). He has been in private practice in integrative medicine for thirty-six years with a focus on integrative oncology and is the author of *Healthy Medicine: A Guide to the Emergence of Sensible, Comprehensive Care* and *Beyond the Medical Meltdown: Working Together for Sustainable Health Care.* Dr. Zieve's work was featured in a chapter in the 2011 book *Defeat Cancer: 15 Doctors of Integrative and Naturopathic Medicine Tell You How.* Dr. Zieve is also the host of Healthy Medicine Radio, interviewing nationally known people in integrative medicine http://healthymedicine.org/html/radio.html.

Glossary

2-Chlorodeoxyadenosine (2CDA)—Also known as cladribine (an antimetabolite), it is a drug used to treat hairy cell leukemia (HCL).

3 plus 7 induction—Chemotherapy regimen consisting of "7+3" (or "3+7"), seven days of cytarabine and three days of an anthracycline.

5-FU—A pyrimidine, typically administered with leucovorin to treat cancers.

Acute lymphoblastic leukemia (ALL)—A form of leukemia with excessive white blood cells known as lymphoblasts.

Acute myelogenous leukemia (AML)—A form of leukemia with excessive cells known as myeloid blasts.

Adenosine deaminase—Also known as ADA, is an enzyme (EC 3.5.4.4) involved in purine metabolism.

Adenosine triphosphate (ATP)—A multifunctional nucleoside triphosphate used in cells as a coenzyme. ATP serves as the principal source of chemical energy within cells for metabolism.

Adriamycin—Also known as doxorubicin, an anthracycline antibiotic closely related to daunomycin, which works by intercalating DNA.

Aesop—A Greek writer credited with a number of popular fables. In many of the tales, animals speak and have human characteristics.

AKT—Also known as Protein Kinase B (PKB), this is a serine/threonine protein kinase that plays a key role in cellular processes such as glucose metabolism, cell proliferation, and apoptosis.

Alpha-ketoglutarate—A metabolic intermediate in the Krebs cycle.

Aminopterin—An antineoplastic drug and immunosuppressive. First used by Sidney Farber, MD, in 1947 to induce remissions in children with leukemia.

Amyotrophic lateral sclerosis—Also known as ALS, this is a form of motor neuron disease caused by the degeneration of upper and lower neurons, located in the ventral horn of the spinal cord and the cortical neurons that provide their efferent input.

Anandamide—A messenger molecule that plays a role in pain, depression, appetite, memory, and fertility. The name is taken from the Sanskrit word *ananda,* meaning "bliss."

Anthocyanins—Any of the many water-soluble red to violet plant pigments related to the flavonoids.

Antioxidant—A molecule capable of inhibiting the oxidation of other molecules. Oxidation reactions can produce free radicals. In turn, these radicals can start chain reactions that cause damage or death to the cell.

Aplasia—A defective development or congenital absence of an organ or tissue.

Apoptosis—The process of programmed cell death (PCD) that may occur in multicellular organisms. These changes include blebbing, cell shrinkage, nuclear fragmentation, chromatin condensation, and chromosomal DNA fragmentation.

ARA-C—Arabinofuranosyl cytidine cytarabine, or cytosine arabinoside, is a chemotherapy agent used mainly in the treatment of acute myeloid leukemia (AML).

Arsenic trioxide—An inorganic compound with the formula As_2O_3 used in the treatment of acute promyelocytic leukemia (APL).

Ascites fluid—An accumulation of fluid in the peritoneal cavity.

Ascorbic acid—The chemical name for vitamin C.

Assay—An examination and determination as to characteristics (as weight, measure, or quality).

All trans retinoic acid (ATRA)—A drug used to treat acne vulgaris and keratosis pilarisis; also used to treat acute promyelocytic leukemia (APL).

ATP—See Adenosine triphosphate.

Atypia—A clinical term for an abnormality in a cell that may be precancerous.

Autoimmune hemolytic anemia (AIHA)—A condition that occurs when antibodies directed against the person's own red blood cells (RBCs) cause them to burst (lyse).

Autotrophs—Meaning *self-feeding*, this is an organism that produces complex organic compounds (such as carbohydrates, fats, and proteins) from simple inorganic molecules.

Avastin—Also known as bevacizumab, this is a monoclonal antibody against VEGF that blocks angiogenesis, the growth of new blood vessels.

Azacytidine—Also known by the trade name Vidaza, 5-azacytidine is a chemical analog of cytidine used in the treatment of myelodysplastic syndrome.

Banting, Frederick—Sir Frederick Grant Banting (1891–1941) was a Canadian medical scientist, doctor, and Nobel laureate noted as one of the main discoverers of insulin.

Bernoulli's principle—Named after the Dutch-Swiss mathematician Daniel Bernoulli who in 1738 published his principle in *Hydrodynamica*; it states that for an inviscid flow, an increase in the speed of the fluid occurs simultaneously with a decrease in pressure.

Best, Charles MD—Dr. Best was a medical scientist and one of the codiscoverers of insulin.

Bevacizumab—See Avastin.

Blast cells—Blast cells are immature precursors of either lymphocytes (lymphoblasts) or granulocytes (myeloblasts). They do not normally appear in peripheral blood.

Blastula—A hollow sphere of cells formed during an early stage of embryonic development.

Bone marrow—The soft, spongy tissue found in the cavities of bones where new blood cells are produced.

Bone marrow transplant—A procedure done to replace damaged or destroyed bone marrow with healthy bone marrow stem cells.

BRCA1, BRCA2—Human genomic fidelity genes that when mutated can result in a hereditary form of breast and ovarian cancer.

CA 19-9—Carbohydrate antigen 19-9, also called cancer antigen 19-9, is a tumor marker used primarily in the management of pancreatic cancer.

CA-125—Cancer antigen 125, or carbohydrate antigen 125, is a tumor marker used primarily to evaluate ovarian cancer treatment.

Caenrhabditis elegans—This free-living, transparent nematode (roundworm) lives in temperate soil environments. It has been used extensively as a model organism for research in molecular biology and has served as an important model in the study of cellular apoptosis.

Calcium channel blockers—These types of drugs block the entry of calcium into the muscle cells of the heart and arteries.

Capecitabine—An oral prodrug of 5-FU used in the treatment of metastatic breast and colorectal cancers.

Carboplatin—A platinum chemotherapy with a reduced toxicity profile used in ovarian, lung, breast, and head and neck cancers. Introduced in the late 1980s, carboplatin is a derivative of the parent compound—cisplatin.

CARET study—The Carotene and Retinol Efficacy Trial (CARET) was a clinical trial of cancer prevention that used beta-carotene in persons at high risk for lung cancer.

Catechins—Flavonoid phytochemical compounds found primarily in green tea, as well in smaller amounts in grapes, black tea, chocolate, and wine, which function as antioxidants.

CD33—A transmembrane protein present on myeloid cells and myeloid precursors.

CEA—Carcinoembryonic antigen is a glycoprotein involved in cell adhesion, usually only produced in a developing fetus, that can be produced by certain cancers of the colon, rectum, breast, ovary, pancreas, and lung.

Cell staining—This technique uses dyes to better visualize cells and cell components under a microscope.

Central dogma—In molecular biology, this principle dictates that the residue-by-residue transfer of sequential information from DNA to RNA to protein is unidirectional.

Cerebellum—Latin for "little brain," a region at the base of the brain that plays an important role in motor control.

Chaperones—In molecular biology, proteins that assist in folding or unfolding and the assembly of macromolecular structures like proteins.

Chemosensitivity testing—A laboratory analysis that uses tumor cells removed from the body and measures the number of cells killed by chemotherapy. A chemosensitivity assay may assist in choosing the best drug or combination for cancer treatment.

CHOP—This is the acronym for a chemotherapy regimen used in the treatment of non-Hodgkin lymphoma consisting of: cyclophosphamide, hydroxydaunorubicin (doxorubicin or Adriamycin), Oncovin (vincristine), and prednisone.

Chromogranin A—A protein found in the blood of patients with carcinoid tumors and other neuroendocrine cancers.

Chronomodulating—Administering chemotherapy treatments and drugs at times that are synchronized with personal biological rhythms.

Cisplatin—Trade name Platinol and Platinol-AQ, a chemotherapy drug widely used to treat numerous cancers with curative impact on germ cell tumors. It was the first member of a class of platinum-containing anticancer drugs, which now also includes carboplatin and oxaliplatin.

Cladribine—See 2-chlorodeoxyadenosine.

Clonogenic assay—This laboratory technique was used to study the effectiveness of specific agents on tumor cell proliferation (clonogenicity). Originally applied in cancer research by Dr. Sydney Salmon, it came to be known as the human stem cell assay. After years of study, it proved unsuccessful for the selection of chemotherapy and has since largely been abandoned.

c-MET—A proto-oncogene that encodes a protein known as hepatocyte growth factor receptor (HGFR) or scatter factor.

Cortisone—A steroid hormone released by the adrenal gland in response to stress. It is used therapeutically for inflammation, autoimmune disease, and the treatment of lymphatic cancer.

Craniotomy—A surgical operation in which a bone flap is temporarily removed from the skull to access the brain.

Crizotinib—An ALK (anaplastic lymphoma kinase) inhibitor, approved for treatment of non-small cell lung cancers (NSCLC) that carry an ALK gene rearrangement.

CyberKnife—A frameless robotic radiosurgery system used to deliver a highly focused radiation beam, often in brain tumors.

Cyproterone acetate—An antiandrogen used in the treatment of metastatic prostate cancer.

Cysteine—A sulfur containing amino acid and constituent of glutathione.

Cytokines—Small signaling protein molecules secreted by the immune system as intercellular communications.

Cytoxan—Cyclophosphamide, a nitrogen mustard alkylating agent, widely used in the treatment of cancer.

Deep venous thrombosis (DVT)—A blood clot (thrombus) in a deep vein.

Density centrifugation—A laboratory procedure used to isolate cells based upon their density.

Dexamethasone—A very potent synthetic member of the glucocorticoids (see Cortisone).

Diabetes mellitus—The most common endocrinologic disorder, diabetes is associated with a deficiency of insulin.

DMSO—An organosulfur compound used as a solvent.

DNA—Deoxyribonucleic acid (DNA), found in the nucleus of cells, contains the genetic instructions used in the development and function of most living organisms.

DVT—See deep venous thrombosis.

EGFR—Epidermal growth factor receptor is one of a family of proteins found on the surface of epithelial cells and often overexpressed on cancer cells. When bound by epidermal growth factor, it signals growth and survival.

Embryogenesis—The process by which an embryo forms and develops.

EML4-ALK—One of the gene rearrangements associated with abnormal ALK expression and activity, originally identified in a subset of NSCLC patients, and the target of crizotonib.

Endosymbiosis—The coexistence of living matter where one organism lives within the body or cells of another organism.

Endothelial growth factor—EGF is a signal protein produced by cells that stimulates vasculogenesis and angiogenesis.

Enzyme—A protein (or protein-based molecule) that speeds up (catalyzes) a chemical reaction.

Enzymologist—A scientist who specializes in studying enzymes.

Epidermal growth factor receptor—see EGFR.

Epigenetics—The study of heritable changes in gene function that occur without changes in the sequence of DNA.

Erlotinib—Trade name Tarceva, a member of the "targeted" drug class that inhibits EGFR signaling, used to treat NSCLC, pancreatic cancer, and other types of cancer.

Esophagus—The muscular tube through which food passes from the throat to the stomach.

Estrogen receptor—A protein found inside the cell nucleus that, when bound by estrogen, initiates downstream signaling in hormone responsive tissues; the target of Tamoxifen.

Everolimus—A derivative of rapamycin, this drug belongs to a class of serine-threonine kinase inhibitors known as the mTOR inhibitors, used in kidney, neuroendocrine, and breast cancer.

Flavonoids—Or bioflavonoids, from the Latin word *flavus* meaning "yellow," are polyphenol antioxidants found naturally in plants.

GABA—The acronym for gamma aminobutyric acid, an amino acid that acts as a neurotransmitter in the central nervous system.

Gallic acid—A phenolic acid found in gallnuts, sumac, witch hazel, tea leaves, oak bark, blueberries, and other plants, used in the pharmaceutical industry as a standard for determining the phenol content.

Gastrula—An animal embryo at the stage following the blastula, when it develops into three layers: ectoderm, mesoderm, and endoderm.

Gestation—The carrying of an embryo or fetus inside a uterus.

Glutathione—Also known as GSH, a tripeptide of glutamic acid, cysteine, and glycine that is among the most important antioxidants in the human cell.

Glycolysis—A series of enzyme-activated reactions through which glucose and other sugars are broken down into simpler molecules (lactic acid or pyruvic acid) for use as energy.

Glycosylation—The process by which a carbohydrate is attached to another molecule.

Hashimoto's disease—An autoimmune disease that afflicts the thyroid and other glandular tissues.

Heat maps—Two-dimensional representations of data in which values are represented as colors. In molecular biology these microarray maps are used to highlight gene expression.

Heat shock proteins—Also known as chaperones, this group of proteins protect cells against heat stress and are overexpressed in some tumors. They function in protein synthesis, protecting nascent proteins from digestion.

Hemoglobin—The substance inside red blood cells that binds to oxygen in the lungs and carries it to the tissues.

HER2—A member of the epidermal growth factor receptor family, also known as Neu or ERBB2, is often mutated or overexpressed in breast cancers, and serves as the target for trastuzumab.

Hermaphroditism—A medical term for an intersex condition in which an individual is born with ovarian and testicular tissue.

Heterotrophs—An organism that is unable to synthesize its own food and depends upon food-producing autotrophs for metabolic energy.

Histiocyte—A type of white blood cell; also called a macrophage.

Histones—Alkaline proteins found in eukaryotic cell nuclei that package and organize DNA into structural units called nucleosomes.

Homeostasis—The property of a system that regulates its internal environment to maintain stable and constant conditions.

Human papilloma virus (HPV)—A sexually transmitted infection associated with genital warts and cancers of the cervix, as well as head and neck.

Hydroxychloroquine—An anti-inflammatory drug used in the treatment of malaria with activity against lupus erythematosus and rheumatoid arthritis.

Hypercoagulability—A state where blood clots form faster than normal.

Immune system—Cells, tissues, and organs within an organism that protect against disease.

Immunodeficiency—A failure of the immune system to adequately protect the body from infection.

Immunohistochemical—A technique used to identify specific proteins in tissues using antibodies that bind to specific molecules.

Immunosuppressant—Any substance that decreases the body's immune responses.

Insulin-like growth factor receptor—A protein found on the surface of some types of cells that bind to insulin-like growth factor (IGF) causing cells to grow and divide.

INTACT 1 Trial—A Phase III clinical trial that tested gefinitib combined with gemcitabine and cisplatin in lung cancer that did not improve efficacy over gemcitabine and cisplatin alone.

INTACT 2 Trial—A Phase III trial that tested gefitinib in combination with paclitaxel and carboplatin in lung cancer that showed no added benefit compared with paclitaxel and carboplatin alone.

Interferon—Naturally occurring proteins made and secreted by cells of the immune system in response to pathogens such as viruses, bacteria, parasites, or tumor cells.

Intraperitoneally—Delivering an injection or infusion directly into the peritoneum, the thin membrane that lines the walls of the abdominal cavity.

Journal of Medicinal Food—peer-reviewed international journal published by Marianne Liebert Publishing that delivers original research on the chemistry and biochemistry of the bioactive constituents of food.

King, Mary Claire PhD—Professor at the University of Washington where she studied interactions between genetics and environmental influences. King is known for the description of the BRCA genes associated with familial breast and ovarian cancer.

Krebs cycle—A sequence of reactions through which most living cells generate energy during the process of aerobic respiration.

Kushi, Michio—Born in Japan in 1926, he helped introduce modern macrobiotics to the United States in the early 1950s.

Lactate dehydrogenase—An enzyme that converts lactate to pyruvate.

Leukemia—A cancer of the blood or bone marrow characterized by an abnormal increase of immature white blood cells called blasts.

Leukopenia—A decrease in the number of white blood cells (leukocytes) found in the blood that places individuals at increased risk of infection.

Liebert, Mary Ann—Founder of Mary Ann Liebert Publishing Company in 1980. The company publishes peer-reviewed academic journals, books, and trade magazines in the areas of biotechnology.

Li-Fraumeni syndrome—A rare disorder caused by the loss of P53 tumor suppressor gene that greatly increases the risk of developing cancer.

Limonene—A cyclic monoterpene found in plants like lemon peel, orange oil, pine needles, and peppermint.

Lou Gehrig's disease—Named after the famous American baseball player, amyotrophic lateral sclerosis (ALS) is a form of motor neuron disease.

Lymphoma—A cancer that arises in the lymphocytes, cells that normally function to protect the body against pathogens as part of the immune system.

Macleod, John James Ricard MD—Collaborated with Frederick Banting and Charles Best in the discovery of insulin, for which Banting and Macleod were jointly awarded the Nobel Prize for Physiology or Medicine in 1923.

Macrobiotics—A dietary regimen that involves eating grains as a staple food supplemented with local vegetables, avoiding highly processed, refined foods and most animal products. Macrobiotics also addresses the manner of eating, stressing the balance of foodstuffs using yin and yang.

Macrophages—Macrophages (from the Greek *makros* ["large"] + *phagein* ["eat"]) are cells produced by the differentiation of monocytes. Monocytes and macrophages are phagocytes.

Malignant—Tending to become worse and/or to cause death. A term used to describe cancer.

Margulis, Lynn PhD—An American biologist and professor at the University of Massachusetts, Amherst, best known for her theory on the origin of eukaryotic organelles known as endosymbiosis.

Mastectomy—Surgical removal of one or both breasts, partially or completely. Mastectomy is usually done to treat breast cancer.

m-BACOD—A second generation combination chemotherapy regimen for lymphoma consisting of methotrexate, bleomycin, doxorubicin, cyclophosphamide, vincristine, and dexamethasone.

MCAT—The Medical College Admission Test.

MEK/ERK—A chain of proteins in the cell that communicates signals from a receptor on the surface of the cell to the nucleus.

Mendel, Gregor—Austrian scientist and Augustinian friar who gained fame posthumously as the founder of the new science of genetics.

Metabolism—The complex physical and chemical processes involved in the maintenance of life.

Metabolomics—The scientific study of chemical processes involving metabolites, metabolism, and the enzymotology of energy production.

Metazoan—Any animal having a body made up of differentiated cells arranged in tissues and organs.

Methylxanthines—Chemical species found in coffee and chocolate that functions as stimulants and bronchodilators.

Micro molar—A concentration of one millionth of a mole per liter.

Microspheroid—Term applied to small clusters of cells that form aggregates, used in the study of human tissues in culture.

Missense mutation—In genetics, a mutation (nonsynonymous) in which a single nucleotide is changed, resulting in a codon that codes for a different amino acid.

Mitochondria—A membrane-enclosed cellular organelle found in eukaryotes, sometimes described as the "cellular power plants" that generate adenosine triphosphate (ATP) used for energy.

Mitosis—The process by which eukaryotic cells separate and divide into two distinct cells, each with a full complement of nuclear DNA.

Monoclonal antibody—Monospecific antibodies that are identical, derived from immune cells that are cloned from a single parent cell, often used to target specific proteins in therapy.

MOPP—The original chemotherapy combination developed for the treatment of advanced Hodgkin disease, consisting of Mustargen, Oncovin, procarbazine, and prednisone.

Morula—An embryo at an early stage of development consisting of cells in a solid ball.

MRI—Magnetic resonance imaging is an imaging test that uses powerful magnets and radio waves to create pictures of the body. It does not use radiation.

mTOR—Mammalian target of rapamycin, known as the mechanistic target of rapamycin; mTOR is a serine/threonine protein kinase that regulates cell growth, proliferation, motility, and survival.

Müllerian duct—Müllerian ducts are paired ducts of the embryo that develop to form the Fallopian tubes, uterus, cervix, and the upper two-thirds of the vagina; in the male, they are lost.

Mustards (nitrogen mustard)—A class of cytotoxic vesicant chemical warfare agents found to possess anticancer properties that developed into the class of drugs known as alkylators.

Myelodysplasia—A group of disorders in which the bone marrow does not function normally and produces an insufficient number of normal blood cells, which can transform into acute leukemia.

Narcan (naloxone)—An opioid antagonist used to counteract the effects of opiate overdose.

Neuron-specific enolase—An enzyme found in neuroendocrine tumors that can be used as a tumor marker.

Neutrinos—Electrically neutral, weakly interacting elementary subatomic particles with a half-integer spin and a disputed but small nonzero mass, able to pass through ordinary matter unaffected.

NF-kB—Nuclear factor kappa-light-chain-enhancer of activated B cells, is a protein complex that controls the transcription of DNA, associated with cellular response to stress, cytokines, free radicals, ultraviolet irradiation, oxidized LDL, and bacterial or viral antigens.

Nitric oxide—Also known as nitrogen monoxide, a binary molecule with the chemical formula NO. It is a free radical and is an important intermediate in the chemical industry, with important biological functions associated with vascular tone.

Nitrogen mustard—See Mustards.

NSCLC—Non-small cell lung cancer.

Nucleotide—Molecules that join together to make up the structural units of RNA and DNA. In addition, nucleotides participate in cellular signaling (cGMP and cAMP), and function in cellular energy (ATP and GTP).

Oncogene addicted—A term coined by I. Bernard Weinstein to describe cancer cell dependence upon specific driver mutations that provide survival advantage and provides the rationale for molecular targeted therapy.

Oophorectomy—Surgical removal of an ovary or ovaries.

Otto, Warburg—German physiologist, medical doctor, and Nobel laureate who described the phenomenon of aerobic glycolysis, now felt to be fundamental to cancer cell physiology.

Oxidative phosphorylation—A metabolic process through which energy is released by the oxidation of nutrients to produce adenosine triphosphate (ATP).

p53—A tumor suppressor protein encoded by the TP53 gene, in which mutations result in a predisposition to cancer.

Paclitaxel—See Taxol.

Panavir R—A proprietary formulation of a lipophilic antioxidant developed by Dr. Sheldon Hendler and Vyrex Corporation as a therapy for AIDS.

Pauling, Linus—An American biochemist, peace activist, author, educator, and recipient of two Nobel prizes.

Pentostatin—Also known as deoxycoformycin, a purine analog that inhibits the enzyme adenosine deaminase used in the treatment of hairy cell leukemia and lymphomas.

Peroxisome—Organelles found in eukaryotic cells involved in the catabolism of long chain fatty acids, branched chain fatty acids, D-amino acids, and polyamines

PET scan—Positron emission tomography (PET) is a nuclear medicine imaging technique that produces images that reflect metabolic activity as measured by the uptake of F18 glucose.

P-glycoprotein—Also known as multidrug resistance protein 1 (MDR1), this membrane efflux pump is a member of the ABC transmembrane transporter proteins, responsible for drug resistance in some tumors.

Phlebitis—Inflammation of a vein, usually in the legs, associated with the formation of blood clots.

PI3K—Phosphatidylinositol 3-kinases (PI 3-kinases or PI3Ks) are a family of enzymes involved in signal transduction associated with cell growth, proliferation, differentiation, and survival.

Piceid—A stilbenoid glucoside and resveratrol derivative found in grapes and *Polygonum cuspidatum.*

Piezoelectric effect—The charge that accumulates in solid materials (crystals, ceramics, and biological matter like bone, DNA, and proteins) in response to applied mechanical stress.

PKC—Protein kinase C, also known as PKC, is a family of protein kinases that control cell functions through the phosphorylation of serine and threonine amino acid residues.

Pluripotent cells—Cells with the ability to differentiate into more than one cell type—e.g., stem cells.

Polyphenols—A structural class of natural, synthetic, and semisynthetic organic chemicals characterized by the presence of multiple phenol structural units.

PR (progesterone receptor)—An intracellular steroid receptor that binds progesterone, encoded by a single PGR gene residing on chromosome 11q22; it has two main forms, A and B, which differ in their molecular weight.

Prednisone—A synthetic form of corticosteroid, more potent than hydrocortisone, used in the treatment of inflammatory conditions, lymphoblastic leukemia, and lymphomas.

Procrustes—In Greek mythology, Procrustes, or "the stretcher" (who hammers out the metal), was a rogue smith and bandit who physically attacked people by stretching them or cutting off their legs, so as to force them to fit the size of an iron bed, known as the Procrustean bed.

Progesterone—A C-21 steroid hormone involved in the female menstrual cycle, pregnancy (supports gestation), and embryogenesis.

PROMACE-CYTABOM—A polychemotherapy regimen for lymphoma consisting of cyclophosphamide, doxorubicin, etoposide, Cytosar, bleomycin, vincristine, methotrexate, and prednisone.

Promyelocytic leukemia—A subtype of acute myelogenous leukemia (AML) known as acute promyelocytic leukemia, associated with the T15-17 translocation that responds to all trans retinoic acid (ATRA) therapy.

Protease inhibitors—A class of drugs used to treat viruses, including HIV and hepatitis C.

Protein kinase C inhibitors—Drugs that inhibit protein kinase C (PKC) activity.

PSA—Prostatic specific antigen, a protein secreted by prostate tissue used to diagnose and monitor prostate cancer in patients.

Pulmonary metastases—Spread of cancer to the lung.

Pyrrhic—From the Greek victory at Asculum (279 BC) that resulted in such devastating costs that the victor Pyrrhus could not fight again, thereby losing to the Romans.

Pyruvate kinase—An enzyme involved in glycolysis that catalyzes the transfer of a phosphate group from phosphoenolpyruvate (PEP) to ADP, yielding pyruvate and one molecule of ATP.

Quercetin—A plant-derived flavonoid found in fruits, vegetables, leaves, and grains. It also may be used as an ingredient in supplements, beverages, or foods, and has anticancer and anti-inflammatory properties.

RAF—A proto-oncogene serine/threonine-protein kinase enzyme that participates in RAS-related cellular signals for survival and proliferation.

Rapamycin—Also known as sirolimus, an immunosuppressant drug used to prevent rejection in organ transplantation that provides survival signals in some malignancies.

RAS—A family of related proteins known as GTPases, commonly mutated in human cancers with potent survival, proliferation, growth, and metastasis-related potential.

Renal cell carcinoma—A type of kidney cancer that starts in the lining of very small tubes (tubules) in the kidney.

Resveratrol—A stilbenoid, natural phenol, and a phytoalexin found in grapes, Chinese gooseberry, and other plants with anticancer properties.

Retinoids—Chemical compounds structurally related to vitamin A that regulate epithelial cell growth.

Rhuematoid arthritis—A chronic autoimmune disease associated with inflammation of the joints and surrounding tissues.

Rothko, Mark (1903–1970)—A Russian-American abstract painter.

SAHA—Subroyl anilide hydroxamic acid is a histone-deacetylase inhibitor sold commercially as vorinostat, used in the treatment of T-cell lymphoma.

Sarcoma—A malignant tumor that arises from mesodermal cells in connective tissues.

Schleiden, Matthia Jakob (1804–1881)—A German botanist and cofounder of the cell theory, along with Theodor Schwann and Rudolf Virchow.

Schwann, Theodore (1810–1882)—A German physiologist, discoverer of Schwann cells, and developer of the cell theory of biology.

SELECT Study—Selenium and Vitamin E Cancer Prevention Trial was a chemoprevention trial designed to test whether these dietary supplements could prevent prostate cancer.

Severe combined immunodeficiency—SCID is an immune system disorder that compromises antibody and T-cell functions resulting in complete loss of protection against infection; known as "bubble boy" disease.

Sexual dimorphism—The phenotypic difference between males and females of the same species.

Simvastatin—See Zocor.

Small interfering RNAs—This is a class of hairpin double-strand RNA molecules (siRNA or silencing RNA) that downregulate mRNA function by binding through nucleotide complementation.

SNP—Single-nucleotide polymorphism is a DNA sequence variation occurring when a single nucleotide in the genome differs between paired chromosomes in an individual.

Solipsist—A philosophical belief that only one's own mind, alone, is sure to exist. Extreme self-centeredness.

Sonic hedgehog—SHH is one of three proteins in the mammalian signaling pathway family called hedgehog and associated with differentiation and stem cell biology.

Sorafenib—Marketed as Nexavar, a drug approved for the treatment of kidney cancer and liver cancer with activity against vascular endothelial growth factor and RAF.

Splice variant—Alternative splicing is a process by which exons of

RNA produced by transcription of a gene are reconnected in multiple ways during RNA splicing.

Stem cells—Cells found in multicellular organisms that can divide (through mitosis) and differentiate into diverse specialized cell types and have the capacity of self renewal.

Stilbenes—Diarylethene hydrocarbons consisting of a transethene double bond substituted with a phenyl group on both carbon atoms of the double bond.

Streptomyces—The largest genus of Actinobacteria and the type genus of the family Streptomycetaceae. Over 500 species of Streptomyces bacteria have been described.

Sunitinib—Marketed as Sutent, an oral, multitargeted receptor tyrosine kinase (RTK) inhibitor used in the treatment of renal cell carcinoma, GIST, and neuroendocrine tumors.

Sutton's law—Borrowed from the bank robber Willie Sutton, who when asked why he robbed banks said, "Because that is where the money is." The phrase is used as a suggestion to not miss the obvious.

Symbiosis—From Ancient Greek *syn* ("with") and *bísis* ("living") is the close and often long-term interaction between different biological species.

Synergy—Two or more things functioning together to produce a result not independently obtainable; supra-additivity.

Systemic lupus erythematosus—SLE or lupus, is a systemic autoimmune disease that affects multiple organs including kidney, skin, lung, and brain.

T and B cells—Subcategories of lymphocytes named for thymus (T) and bursa (B) as their tissues of origin.

Taxol—Generic name paclitaxel, a microtubule inhibitor used in cancer chemotherapy, extracted from the bark of the Pacific yew tree (*Taxus brevifolia*).

Telomerase—A DNA polymerase that is a ribonucleoprotein that catalyzes the elongation of chromosomal telomeres in eukaryotic cells and is particularly active in cancer cells.

Temsirolimus—A synthetic derivative of rapamycin, a kinase inhibitor.

Theobroma cacao—A South American evergreen tree of the Sterculiaceae family that produces cocoa beans from which chocolate is extracted.

Theobromine—Also known as xantheose, a bitter alkaloid of the cacao plant, found in chocolate and other foods, including the leaves of the tea plant and the kola (or cola) nut.

Thiols—An organosulfur compound that contains carbon-bonded sulfhydryl groups.

Thoracotomy—A surgical exploration of the lung.

Thymidine phosphorylase—An enzyme that catalyzes the chemical reaction of thymidine + phosphate to thymine + 2-deoxy-alpha-D-ribose 1-phosphate; responsible for the activation of capecitabine (Xeloda).

Topoisomerase 2—An enzyme that controls and alters the topologic states of DNA during transcription.

Trans fatty acids—The common name for an unsaturated fat with *trans*-isomer fatty acid(s).

Trousseau, Armand (1801–1867)—A French internist who diagnosed migratory thrombophlebitis in himself as a diagnostic finding associated with pancreatic cancer.

Urea cycle—The major end product of nitrogen metabolism in humans and mammals allowing the removal of ammonia, the product of oxidative deamination reactions.

Vascular endothelial growth factor (VEGF)—A signal protein produced by cells that stimulate vasculogenesis and angiogenesis.

VEGF—See Vascular endothelial growth factor.

Vemurafenib—Also known as PLX4032, is a selective inhibitor of the enzyme B-Raf upregulated in malignant melanoma and specifically active against the V600E mutant subtype.

Vinblastine—An antimicrotubule drug used to treat certain kinds of cancer, including Hodgkin lymphoma, non-small cell lung cancer, breast cancer, head and neck cancer, and testicular cancer.

Vinorelbine—Trade name Navelbine, is an antimitotic chemotherapy drug that is given as a treatment for some types of cancer, including breast cancer and non-small cell lung cancer.

Virchow, Rudoph (1821–1902)—A German pathologist and biologist considered "the father of modern pathology."

Wolffian duct—Also known as the mesonephric duct, a paired organ found in mammals, including humans, during embryogenesis, that serves as the anlage male reproductive organs.

Wyeth Pharmaceuticals—An American pharmaceutical company acquired by Pfizer Corporation in 2009.

Xocolatl—Aztec term for chocolate.

Zocor—Generic name simvastatin, a statin drug used to control elevated cholesterol in patients with hypercholesterolemia.

References

Chapter 2: A Brief History of Chemotherapy and Chemosensitivity Testing

Black, M. M. and Spear, F. D. 1954. Further observations on the effects of cancer chemotherapeutic agents on the in vitro dehydrogenase activity of cancer tissue. *J Natl Cancer Inst* 14:1147–1158.

Krumbhaar, E. B. and Krumbhaar, H. D. 1919. The blood and bone marrow in yelloe[w] cross gas (mustard gas) poisoning: Changes produced in the bone marrow of fatal cases. *J Med Res* 40(3):497–508.3.

Salmon, S. E., Hamburger, A. W., Soehnlen, B. S., et al. 1978. Quantitation of differential sensitivity of human tumor stem cells to anticancer drugs. *N Engl J Med* 298:1321–1327.

Selby, P., Buick, R. N., and Tannock, I. 1983. A critical appraisal of the "human tumor stem-cell assay." *N Engl J Med* 20:308(3):129–134.

Chapter 3: Early Scientific Discoveries

Nagourney, R. A., Evans, S. S., Messenger, J. C., et al. 1993. 2 Chlorodeoxyadenosine activity and cross resistance patterns in primary cultures of human hematologic neoplasms. *Br J Cancer* 67(1):10–14.

Nagourney, R. A., Jacobson, R. J., Woolley, and P. V. 1984. Accurate prediction of response to treatment in human leukemia utilizing a vital-dye exclusion chemosensitivity technique. *Proc Am Soc Clin Oncol* 208 (abstr.).

Nagourney, R. A., Weisenthal, L. M., and Kern, D. H. 1990. In vitro detection of high grade drug resistance in fresh specimens of human non-small cell lung cancer: Rational selection of chemotherapy based upon patterns of high grade resistance. *Proc Amer Assoc Canc Res* 31:361, 2137 (abstr.).

Woolley, P. V., Von Hoff, D. D., Kyle, G. W., et al. 1986. Biology of colon cancer resistance to treatment. In *Biology and treatment of colorectal cancer metastases*, A. J. Mastromarino (Ed.). Boston: Martinus Nijhoff.

Chapter 12: East Meets West

Nagourney, R. A., Evans, S. S., Messenger, J. C., et al. 1993. 2-Chloro-deoxyadenosine activity and cross-resistance patterns in primary cultures of human hematologic neoplasms. *Br J Cancer* 67:10–14.

Chapter 13: Garlic, Wine, Chocolate, and More

Lippman, S. M., Klein, E. A., Goodman, P. J., et al. 2009. Effect of selenium and vitamin E on risk of prostate cancer and other cancers: the Selenium and Vitamin E Cancer Prevention Trial (SELECT). *JAMA* 301(1):39–51.

Mei, X. 1982. Garlic and gastric cancer: the influence of garlic on the level of nitrate and nitrite in gastric juice. *Acta Nutr Sin* 4:53–56.

Moreno-Labanda, J. F., Mallavia, R., Perez-Fons, L., et al. 2004. Determination of piceid and resveratrol in Spanish wines deriving from Monastrell (Vitis vinifera L.) grape variety. *J Agric Food Chem.* 52(17):5396–5403.

Omenn, G. S., Goodman, G. E., Thornquist, M. D., et al. 1996. Risk factors for lung cancer and for intervention effects in CARET, the Beta-Carotene and Retinol Efficacy Trial. *J Natl Cancer Inst.* 88(21):1550–1559.

Chapter 14: Treatable Cancers Should Be Treated Correctly

Martin, M., Piefkowski, T., Mackey, J., et al. 2005. Adjuvant docetaxel for node-positive breast cancer. *N Engl J Med* 352:2302–2313.

Nagourney, R. A., Link, J. S., Blitzer, J. B., et al. 2000. Gemcitabine plus cisplatin repeating doublet therapy in previously treated, relapsed breast cancer patients. *J Clin Oncol* 18(11):2245–2249.

Chapter 15: When All Else Fails

Kroep, J. R., Peters, G. J., and Nagourney, R. A. 2006. Clinical activity of gemcitabine as a single agent and in combination. In *Deoxynucleoside analogs in cancer therapy*, J. Peters Godefridus, PhD (Ed.). Totowa, NJ: Humana Press Publishers.

Chapter 18: What to Do When Your Genes Don't Fit

Brewer, C. A., Sommers, B. L., Evans, S. S., et al. 2008. Capecitabine plus vinorelbine: An active drug combination with evidence of synergy and sequence dependence. Proc Amer Assoc for Canc Res, 2811.

Gad, S., Scheuner, M. T., Pages-Berhouet, S., et al. 2001. Identification of a large rearrangement of the BRCA1 gene using colour bar code on combed DNA in an American breast/ovarian cancer family previously studied by direct sequencing. *Journal of Medical Genetics* 38(6):388–392.

Poliseno, L., Salmena, L., Zhang, J., et. al. 2010. A coding-independent function of gene and pseudogene mRNAs regulates tumour biology. *Nature* 465:1033–1038.

Watson, J. D. and Crick, F. H. C. 1953. Molecular structure of nucleic acids: A structure for deoxyribose nucleic acid. *Nature* 171:737–738.

Chapter 20: Targeted Therapies

Nagourney, R. A., Chow, C., Su, Y. Z., et al. 2002. Activity of ZD1839 (Iressa) alone and combined with cytotoxic rdugs in human tumor primary cultures. *Proc Amer Assoc Canc Res* 43:787, 3902 (abstr.).

Appendix A: Cancer Research Explained

Djulbegovic, B., Kumar, A., and Soares, H. P. 2006. What is the probability that new cancer treatments are better than standard treatments? Proceedings of the American Society of Clinical Oncology 6120 (abstr.).

Roberts, T. G. Jr., Lynch, T. J. Jr., and Chabner, B. A. 2003. The phase III trial in the era of targeted therapy: unraveling the "go or no go" decision. *J Clin Oncol.* 21(19):3683–3695.

Soares, H. P., Djulbegovic, B., Kumar, A., Tanvetyanon, T., and Bepler, G. 2006. Evaluation of publicly sponsored lung cancer trials in US: Are experimental treatments better than the control ones? Proceedings of the American Society of Clinical Oncology 7157 (abstr.).

Appendix B: What to Expect When You're Expecting a Conversation with Your Oncologist

Ferro, S. A., Myer, B. S., Wolff, D. A., et al. 2008. Variation in the cost of medications for the treatment of colorectal cancer. *Am J Manag Care* 14(11):717–25 (abstr.).

Appendix C: A Practical Guide for the Use of Chemosensitivity Testing

Bookman, M. A., Brady, M. F., Mcguire, W. P., et al. 2009. Evaluation of new platinum-based treatment regimens in advanced-stage ovarian cancer: A phase III trial of the Gynecologic Cancer InterGroup. *JCO* 27(9):1419–1425.

Index

A

Acetate groups, 122
Acquired immunodeficiency
    syndrome. *See* AIDS.
Actinomycin D, 175
Active vs inactive drugs, 91–92
Acupressure, 28, 73
Acupuncture, 28, 73
Acute lymphoblastic leukemia.
    See ALL.
Acute myelogenous leukemia,
    16–17
Acute promyelocytic leukemia.
    See APL.
Adenosine deaminase, 18
Adenosine triphosphate. *See* ATP.
Adrenal gland, 61, 63
Adriamycin, 81–83, 177
ADVANCES in Cancer Treatment,
    193
Advocacy, clinical, 194
Aerobic glycosis, 111
Aesop, 1, 4

AIDS, 161–163
Akbarpour, Ferre, 189
AKT, 19
ALK gene mutation, 131–132
Alkylating agents, 19
All Trans Retinoic Acid. *See*
    ATRA.
ALL, 47–48
Allen, Sue, 139–146
Allopathic medicine, 28
Allyl sulfides, 74
Alopecia, 82
Alpha-interferon, 16, 37
Alpha-ketoeglutarate, 111
ALS, 161
American Association for Cancer
    Research, 24, 39, 136, 138,
    167
American Consul General,
    Barbados, 16–17
American Society of Clinical
    Oncology, 17, 20, 96, 136
Ames test, 159

Ames, Bruce, 159
Aminopterin, 2
AML. *See* Acute myelogenous
     leukemia.
Amoebas, 108
AMP kinase, 30–31
Amyotrophic lateral sclerosis.
     See ALS.
Amytal, 149
Anandamine, 76–77
Andrews Air Force Base, 16
Anklyosing spondylitis, 27
Anthocyanins, 74
Anthracyclines, 83
Antibodies, 45
Antimycin A., 149
Antioxidants, 30, 68, 76
Antivascular therapies, 104
APL, 51
Apoptosis. 37, 40–41, 43–46, 48,
     49, 76, 158, 160–161. *See also*
     Cells, Death.
Arabinofuranosyl cytidine. *See*
     ARA-C.
ARA-C, 16–17
Aromatherapy, 28, 73
Arsenic trioxide, 149
Assay criteria, 185–188
AstraZeneca, 137
Atherosclerotic disease, 160
ATP, 30, 149, 156, 158
ATRA, 53
Atwood, Linette, 52–55
Atwood, Wayne, 51–55
Autoimmune diseases, 27, 160
Autotrophs, 156
Avastin, 104
Ayurvedic medicines, 28

Azacytidine, 122
AZD1839. *See* Itessa.

B

Baker, James, 21
Banting, Frederick, 157
B-cell leukemia, 19
B-cell non-Hodgkin lymphoma,
     162
Beltsville, Maryland, 97–101
Bendamustine, 71
Best, Charles, 157
Beta-carotene, 77
Bethesda North Hospital,
     Cincinnati, 89
Bevacizumab, 104, 176, 177
Beyond the Medical Meltdown:
     Working Together for
     Sustainable Health Care, 195
Biochemistry, 111
Bio-Medical Center, Tijuana,
     Mexico, 69
Biotech companies, 21
Blast cells, 48, 53
Blayney, Douglas, 96
Blitzer, Jonathan, 52
Block Center for Integrative
     Cancer Treatment, 190
Block, Keith, 32, 189–190
Block, Penny, 190
Blood vessels, 160–161
Blood-brain barrier, 143
B-lymphocytes, 18
Bone marrow, 2–3, 9, 116, 186
     aplasia, 9
     transplants, 17, 54
Boston University, 7, 223
Boyd, D. Barry, 190

BRAF, 150
Brain tumors, 143
BRCA1 gene mutation, 113, 115
BRCA2 gene mutation, 113, 115
Breast cancer, 2–3, 29, 80–83,
    113–116, 119, 128, 168, 175,
    176
  drugs for, 177–178
Bristol-Myers Squibb, 167
Brookings Institute, 100
Burt, Shari, 89

C
Caffeine, 76
Calcium channel blockers, 21
CAM, 28, 73
Cancer Decisions Newsletter, 193
Cancer Decisions, 193
Cancer Guide Consultations,
    191
Cancer Research, 49
Cancer, ix–x, 1–4, 5–13, 15–25,
    27–33, 35–37, 39–42, 43–46,
    47–50, 51–55, 57–59, 61–66,
    67–72, 73–78, 79–87, 89–101,
    103–108, 109–112, 113–128,
    129–133, 135–146, 147–150,
    151–156, 157–164. *See also*
    types of Cancer such as
    Breast; Colon; Lung;
    Ovarian, etc.
  alternative treatments, 32
  causes of, 151–156
  environmental factors in,
    153–154
  prognostication, 79–80
  research, 112, 118–120,
    147–150, 165–168

  standard care, 172–173
  testing, 182–183, 185–188
  therapies, 127–128, 135–146,
    172–174, 182–183
Cannabinoids, 76
Capecitabine, 114–115, 159,
    177–179
Carboplatin, 61, 63, 89, 92, 137,
    141, 176, 177–178, 179,
    180–181
Carcinogenesis, 44
Cardiovascular disease, 160
CARET Study, 77
Carotenoids, 30
Carroll, Rick, 61–66
Carson, Dennis, 18, 19
Caspases, 40
Catechins, 76
Catecholamines, 31
CD33, 53
CD4-positive cells, 162
CEA, 142
Cecchi, Gary, 106
Cedars-Sinai Medical Center, 61,
    65, 140
Cell death assays, 172
Cell development, 121–122
Cell dynamics. *See* Homeostais.
Cell phones, 153
Cell separation, 15
Cells,
  death, 36–37, 39–41, 43–47, 49,
    98, 127–128, 138, 152, 158,
    161, 163–164, 170–172, 224
  division, 2–3
  single-cell, 109
Central dogma, 121
Cervical cancer, 151

Cetuximab, 176–177
Chemoresistance, 24
Chemosensitivity testing, 9–13,
      24, 36, 97–101, 183
   guide for use, 175–183
Chemotherapeutics, ix, 21–22
Chemotherapy, 8 , 41, 43, 47,
      53–55, 68–72, 80–83, 89–96,
      103–107, 113–116, 130, 140,
      169, 185
   early scientific discoveries,
      15–25
   history of, 9–13
   testing, 10–13, 185–188
Childhood leukemia, 168
China, 75
Chinese medicine, 28
Chocolate, 74, 76–77
CHOP chemotherapy, 2, 72
Chotiocarcinoma, 175
Chow, Craig, 136
Chronic lymphocytic leukemia.
      See CLL.
Cigarette smoke, 153
Cisplatin, 39, 58, 62–63, 82–83,
      92–94, 106, 114, 132, 137, 141,
      142, 177, 178, 180–181
City of Hope, 84, 142
Cleveland Clinic, 90
Clinical trials (protocols),
      165–168
   phase I, 165–166
   phase II, 166–167
   phase III, 167–168
CLL, 20
Clonogenic assay, 11–13, 36
c-MET, 131, 139
CMP, 183

Cold Spring Harbor, 122
Colon cancer, 23
   drugs for, 176–177
Columbia University School of
      Medicine, 7, 12, 138
Complementary alternative
      medicine. *See* CAM.
Comprehensive Metabolic
      profile. *See* CMP.
Corticosteroids, 47
Costs of therapies, 173–174
Cousins, Norman, 27–28
Cowan, Clyde L., 35
Crizotinib, 130–133, 150, 181
Croce, Carlo, 3
Croxall, Thomas Henry, 1
Cutaneous lymphoma, 122
Cyanide, 149
Cyclophosphamide, 176, 177,
      178–179, 180
Cyproterone acetate, 39
Cysteine, 103
Cytotoxic drugs, 10
Cytoxan, 19–20, 82, 83

D

Dana-Farber Cancer Institute,
      141
Dartmouth College, 37
De Candolle, Alphonse, 75
Deep venous thrombosis. *See*
      DVT.
*Defeat Cancer: 15 Doctors of
      Integrative and Naturopathic
      Medicine Tell You How*, 195
Dehydration, 85
Department of Health and Human
      Services (HHS), 96–97

DES, 154
Descartes, Rene, 37
Deuterostomes, 121
Dexamethasone, 48
Diabetes mellitus, 157, 161
Dick, Cameron, 57–58
Dicke, Karel, 54
Diet, 32, 73–78
Diethylstilbestrol. *See* DES.
Diffusion, 110
DNA, 10, 39, 41, 51, 112 113–128,
     133, 164
  changes to, 152
  code, 121
  gel electrophoresis, 49, 118
  non-coding, 124
  polymerases, 116–117
  viral sequences, 152
Dobkin, Jeff, 115
Docetaxel, 176, 177–179, 181
Doxorubicin, 175, 178, 180
Dreher, Henry, 191
Drug development, 168
Drug resistance, 63–64,171
Drug selections, 176–182
Drug tests, 165–168
Drug-response profiling, 175
Drugs, chemotherapy, 2,
     175–183
Ductal carninoma, 81
DVT, 85

E

E6 protein, 46
E7 protein, 46
Easter Island (Rapa Nui), 147
Eastman, Alan, 37, 39
Eclecticism, 33

EDR. *See* Extreme drug
     resistance.
Efflux pumps, 103
Effusions, malignant, 186
EGFR, 130, 135–136, 139, 142
Electromagnetic radiation, 153
Eli Lilly and Company, 167
EML4-ALK, 139
Endorphins, 30
Endosymbiosis, 109
Ensure, 144
Enzymology, 111
Epidermal growth factor
     receptors. See EGFR.
Epidermal growth factor, 111,
     137, 141
Epigenetics, 122
Erlotinib. *See* Tarceva.
Erythropoietin, 104
Estrogen receptor (ER)-positive
     breast cancer, 80–83
Estrogen, 153–155
Etoposide, 180–181
EuroMed Foundation Integrative
     Cancer Clinic, 194–195
Evans, Steve, 49
Everolimus, 148
Ex Vivo Analysis of Programmed
     Cell Death, 224
Exercise, 30, 32
Extreme drug resistance, 22–24
     assay, 97, 101
     tests, 91

F

FAC, 80
Farber, Sydney, 10
FDA, 136, 163, 166–167

FedEx, 187
Fermi, Enrico, 35
Fiber, dietary, 30
5-FU (drug), 16, 37, 104, 144, 159, 176, 177
5-FU plus Adriamycin plus Cytoxan. *See* FAC.
Flavonoids, 74–75
Flow cytometry, 49
Fludarabine, 20
FOLFIRI, 176–177
FOLFOX, 176, 179
Food, 29, 73–78, 153
Free radicals, 30, 152, 161, 162, 163
Free University of Amsterdam, 93
Freuhauf, John, 100
Friedberg, John, 104–108
Fumarate hydratase, 111
Functional profiling, 223

G
GABA, 68
Gamma amino butyric acid. *See* GABA.
Garlic, 29–30, 73–74
Garon, Edward B., 131
Gastric cancer, 75
Gefitinib. *See* Iressa.
Gemcitabine, 58–59, 61, 63–64, 82–83, 92–94, 106, 114, 132, 137, 141, 142, 177–179, 181
Genentech, 137
Genes, 112, 113–128, 152
Genetica (firm), 90, 99
Genomics, 111–112, 116–128, 148, 164

Georgetown University, ix, 223
 Department of Biochemistry, 7–8
 Lombardi Cancer Center, 5, 15, 17, 32
 Medical School, 8, 12
Gilman, Alfred, 9
Glossary, 197–218
Glucosylation, 126
Glutaminolysis, 111
Glutathione depletors, 21
Glutathione, 103
Glycolysis, 110, 148
GOG-182 trial, 178
Goodman, Louis, 9
Grapes, 75–76
Growth factors, 110

H
Hairy cell leukemia, 19
Hanbidge, David, 58–59
Harbor View Hospital, 21
Harvard University, 10, 122
Hashimoto's disease, 160
Healing arts, 28
Healthy Medicine Academy, 195
Healthy Medicine Radio, 195
Healthy Medicine: A Guide to the Emergence of Sensible, Comprehensive Care, 195
Heat maps, 120
Hemolytic anemia, 106
Hendler, Sheldon S., 67, 73, 162–164
Hepatitis C, 61
Hepatocyte growth factor, 111
HER2, 81–83, 139, 177
Herbs, 67

Herceptin, 83
HIV, 162
Hodgkin disease, 8
Homoestasis, 3
Horn, Marcia K., 191
Horvitz, Robert, 3, 40
Hospice, 61–66
Hoxsey formula, 69
Human epidermal growth factor
    receptor2. *See* HER2.
Human genome project, 117,
    121
Human immunodeficiency
    virus. *See* HIV.
Human papilloma virus (HPV),
    46, 151
Human tumor chemosensitivity,
    15
Human tumor stem cell assay.
    See Salmon assay.
Hydrogen peroxide, 153
Hydroxychloroquine, 142
Hyperglycemia, 157

I
IDEAL I and II trials, 136
Ifosfamide, 180
IGFR, 135, 130
Immune system, 18, 153,
    160–161
Infectious diseases, 44
Inflammation, 32, 76, 153
Insulation potentiation therapy
    (PT), 194
Insulin signaling, 147
Insulin, 157
Insulin-like growth factor
    receptors. *See* IGFR.

Insulin-like growth factor,
    111–112
INTACT I and II trials, 137
Integrative oncologic care, 32
International Cancer Advocacy
    Network, 192
International Drug Resistance
    Symposium, 48
*Introduction to Macrobiotic
    Cooking*, 68
Iressa, 64, 130, 132, 136–138, 141
Irinotecan, 62, 64, 144, 145,
    176–177, 180–181
IROX, 176
Islets of Langerhans, 157

J
Jewish heritage, 113
John Harvey (ship), 9
Johnson, Lyndon B., 117
Journal of Biological Chemistry, 137
Journal of Medicinal Food, 73, 78

K
Kaposi's sarcoma, 162
Kapuler, Alan, 28, 67, 73
Kern, David H., 22–24, 100
Kidney cancer, 103–108
Kidneys, removal of, 107–108
Kiesner, Frank, 100
Kinases, 111
King, Mary Claire, 113
Krebs cycle, 110, 148
Kris, Mark G., 131
Kuper, Ryan, 129–133
Kushi, Aveline, 68
Kushi, Michio, 68, 69, 73
Kyle, Rick, 36

L

Laboratory models, 170
Laboratory-directed therapy,
    questions and answers about,
    169–174
LaLanne, Jack, 108
Lapatinib, 178
Laughter, 27
Laying on of hands, 28
Lemon zest, 77–78
Lennon, John, 155
Leucovorin, 176
Leukemia (journal), 49
Leukemia, 10, 15–16, 49, 79, 149,
    168, 186. *See also* types of
    Leukemia.
    therapy, 17–18
Leukopenia, 9
Liebert, Mary Ann, 73
Life Over Cancer, 190
Lifestyle, 28, 29, 31, 32, 71, 73,
    77, 85
Li-Fraumeni syndrome, 46
Ligases, 125
Limonene, 77–78
Lipids, 119, 160
Lipitor, 161
Liposomal doxorubicin, 178–179
LKB-1, 30
Lockwood, Steve, 84–87
Lodi, Thomas, 192–193
Long Beach Memorial Medical
    Center, 21, 47, 49, 51, 57, 62,
    94
    Pediatric Oncology Group, 47
    Todd Cancer Institute, 62
Lou Gehrig's disease. *See* ALS.

Lumpers, 155, 158–159, 163
Lung cancer, 23–24, 57–59, 79,
    128, 129–133, 136–137,
    139–146, 168
    drugs for, 175, 180–181
Lutein, 30
Lycopene, 30
Lymph nodes, 61–66, 68–72,
    80–83, 144
    biopsies, 105–106
Lymphocytes, 31, 45, 147, 160,
    162
Lymphoma, 2, 15, 18, 79. *See also*
    types of Lymphomas.
    low-grade, 20
Lymphosarcoma, 9

M

M.D. Anderson, Texas, 90
Macleod, J.J.R., 157
Macrobiotics, 68, 73
Macrophages, 160
Magnesium, 30
Maintenance therapies, 86
MammaPrint, 118
Manganese, 30
Margulis, Lynn, 109
Markers, 79
Masectomy, 81
Massachusetts General Hospital,
    132
Massage, 28
m-BACOD, 2
McConnell, Douglas, 58
McGill University, 7, 223
McKenna Jr., Robert, 65
Medicare, 97–101

Meditation, 28, 73
MEK/ERK, 139
Melanoma, 23, 79, 150, 168
Melphalan, 179
Membrane integrity, 49
Memorial Sloan-Kettering
    Cancer Center, 32, 51, 53–54,
    90, 131, 141
Mena, Raul, 130
Mendel, Gregor, 121
Mendelian genetics, 121
Metabolic disorders, 119
Metabolism, 29, 161–164
Metabolomics, 111, 119, 148
Metazoan, 110
Metformin, 29
Methotrexate, 175, 177
Methyl groups, 122
Microspheriod isolation, 15
Mind-Body Unity: A New Vision for
    Mind-Body Science and
    Medicine, 191
Mitochondria, 110, 152
Mono Lake, CA, 149
MOPP, 2
Morich, Dieter, 71
Moss Reports, 32
Moss, Ralph, 32, 193
Moyad, Mark, 29
mRNA, 123–124
mTOR inhibitors, 104
mTOR, 139, 147–148
Murgu, Septimiu Dan, 145
Music, 28
Mustard alkylator, 71
Mustard gas, 9–10
Myelodysplasia, 116

Myelodysplastic syndrome, 122
Myeloid leukemia, 19

N
NAD, 156
Nagourney, Robert A., x, 58–59,
    62, 89, 194
    biography, 223–224
    education, 7–8
NASA, 117–118
Natale, Ronald B., 140
National Cancer Institute, ix, 8,
    11, 166
National Comprehensive Cancer
    Network (NCCN), 172–173
National Gallery of Art,
    Washington, DC, 5
National Surgical Adjuvant
    Breast and Bowel Project,
    167
Nature (journal), 116, 124
Naturopathy, 69, 71
Navelbine, 141, 144, 145
Neurological diseases, 161
Neutrino, 35–37
New England Journal of Medicine,
    11, 36, 48, 78, 131, 166
Newman, G. Nathan, 139
Newsweek, 192
NF-kB, 76
Nitrogen mustard, 2, 43
Nobel Prize, 35, 40, 157, 159
Non-Hodgkin B-cell lymphoma,
    68–72
Non-Hodgkin lymphoma, 8
Non-small-cell lung cancer. *See*
    NSCLC.

Notch, 139
NSCLC, 61–66, 173, 180–181

O
Oaclitaxel, 176
Oasis of Healing, An, 192
Oat cell carcinoma. *See* SCLC.
Ohio State University, Columbus,
    90
Omega-3 fatty acids, 30
Oncogene addicted cells, 138
Oncologists, 2
    questions and answers for,
    169–174
Oncotech, Inc., 21–25, 90–92,
    96–101
Oncotype DX, 118
Oral cavity cancer, 151
Orange County Immune
    Institute, 189
Orange zest, 77–78
Origin of Cultivated Plants, The, 75
Ottesen, Ingrid, 80–83
Ou, Sai-Hong Ignatius, 131–132
Outliving Cancer, 3
Ovarian cancer, 89–101, 113–116,
    128, 168, 176, 178–179
Oxaliplatin, 176
Oxidative phosphorylation, 110

P
P53 gene, 46, 152
Paclitaxel, 177, 178–179, 180–181
Panavir R, 162
Pancreatic cancer, 80, 84–87
Pandolfi, Pier Paolo, 124
Panke, Liz, 89–101

Panke, Thomas, 89–101
Parkinson's disease, 161
Patient Advocacy, 194
Patient Resource Cancer Guide, 55
Pauli, Wolfgang, 35
Pauling, Linus, 78, 159
Peace Seeds repository, 68, 72
Pemetrexed, 176, 181
Pentose shunt, 148
Pentostatin, 19
Peroxidases, 153
Peroxisome, 153
PET/CT scans, 61, 65, 86, 115,
    140, 141, 142, 144
P-glycoprotein, 103
Pharmaceutical Executive, 192
Phenolics, 74
Phlebitis. *See* DVT.
Phosphates, 126
PI3K, 139
Piezoelectric effect, 153
PKC, 139
Platins, 177
Platinum-based therapy, 90, 93,
    115, 141
Polyphenols, 74, 76
Predictive factors, 79–80
Progesterone receptor, 81
Progesterone, 104, 153
PRO-MACE-Cytabom, 2
Prostate cancer, 29, 39, 77
Protein kinase C inhibitors, 21
Proteins, 119, 123–126, 152, 155
    heat shock, 125
Purine analog backones, 71
Purple anthocyanins, 68
Pyruvate kinase, 111

Q

Qigong, 28, 73
Questions and answers about
    laboratory-directed therapy,
    169–174

R

Radenski, Paul, 98
Radiation, 47, 58–59, 96, 143, 144
    CyberKnife, 144, 145
RAF protein, 155
Rapamune, 147
Rapamycin (Sirolimus), 147–148
RAS, protein, 155
Raskin, Jay, 22
Rational Therapeutics (firm), 50,
    55, 61, 89, 105, 182, 185–188,
    193, 223
Red blood cells, 104
Reed, John, 3
References, 219–222
Renal cell carcinoma. *See* Kidney
    cancer.
Renneker, Mark, 193–194
Resources, 189–195
Resveratrol, 75–76
Retinoblastoma protein, 152
Retinoids, 51
Retroperitoneal space, 63, 71
Rheumatoid arthritis, 160
Ribonucleic acid. *See* RNA.
RNA, 123–126, 162, 164
    polymerases, 116–117
    small interfering, 123–125
Rockefeller University, 67
Rogers, Will, 75
Rosemary, 30

Rosenberg, Steven, ix, 63
Rotenone, 149
Rothschild Institute, Paris, 67
Royal Victoria Hospital,
    Montreal, 31
Ruehlman, Peter, 89–90, 93–95

S

SAHA, 122
Salmon assay, 11–12
Salmon, Sidney, 11–12
Salvador, Evelyn, 83
Salvage regimen, 62, 90
Sanchez, Robert, 162
Sarcoma, soft tissue, ix
Saturday Review, The, 27
Schein, Philip S., 8, 20
Schleiden, Matthias Jakob, 1
Schwann, Theodor, 1
SCID, 18
SCLC, 57–59, 168, 180
Scripps Institute, 18–20, 67, 70,
    223
Seahorse X Extracellular Flux
    Analyzer, 150
SELECT Study, 77
Selenium, 30, 77
Self-antigens, 160
Selye, Hans, 31
Sensitivity tests, 182–183
Sepulveda Veteran's
    Administration, 22
Serine, 126
Severe combined
    immunodeficiency. *See* SCID.
Sexual dimorphism, 44
Shuman, Robert, 62, 66

Silicon chips, 120
Silverstein, Melvin J., 80–81
Single agent alkylators, 177
Single-nucleotide polymorphism,
    158
Slamon, Dennis, 81
Small Business Innovation
    Research, 21
Small cell lung cancer. *See* SCLC.
SmithKline, 22
Smulson, Mark, 7–8
SOD, 161
Solis, Diana, 94
Sonic hedgehog, 139
Sorafenib, 104
Specificity tests, 182–183
Specimens,
    quantities, 186
    sending, 186–187
Spices, 30
Spiegelman, Sol, 12
Splitters, 155, 158–159, 163
Spontaneous Healing, 69
Squamous cell carcinoma, 143
St. Joseph's Medical Center,
    Burbank, CA, 129
Staining techniques, 49
Standard care, 172–173
Statins, 29, 161
Stem cells, 12
    transplants, 54
Steroid hormones, 153–155
Stevens Steak and Seafood
    House, Los Angeles, 108
Stilbenes, 74
Stress, 31, 32
Stritter, Gwendolyn, 194

Sun Tzu, 12
Sunitinib, 104, 150
Superoxide dismutase. *See* SOD.
Surgery, 113
Sutent, 104
Synergy, 16, 36–37
Systemic lupus erythematosus
    (SLE), 160
Szent-Györgyi, Albert, 149

T
TAC, 80
TAH-BSO, 89
Talc granuloma, 65–66
TALENT trail, 137
Tamoxifen, 80
Tarceva, 64, 130, 136, 137, 141,
    142, 150, 181
Taxanes, 177
Taxol, 89, 92, 137, 141, 145, 161,
    177–178
Taxotere plus Adriamycin plus
    Cytoxan. *See* TAC.
T-cell leukemia, 19
T-cell lymphoma, 19
T-cells, 18–19
TEAC, 30
Telomerase, 76
Temsirolimus, 148
Testosterone, 153–154
Tests, sensitivity vs specificity,
    182–183
Tew, Kenneth, 15
Therapies, targeted, 135–146, 150
    questions and answers about,
    169–174
    testing, 182–183

Thiamin, 30
Thiols, 74
Thiosulfinates, 74
Thoracentesis, 70
Thoracotomies, ix, 65, 130
Threonine, 126
Thymidine phosphorylase, 37, 159
Tissue, human, 127
T-lymphocytes, 18
Topotecan, 58–59, 89, 92, 179, 180
Total abdominal hysterectomy and bilateral oophorectomy. *See* TAH-BSO.
Toxicities, 2, 10–11
Toxins, 103
Trans fatty acids, 153
Trastuzumab, 177–178
TRIBUTE trial, 137
TriHealth System, Cincinnato, 90
Trolox equivalent antioxidant capacity. *See* TEAC.
Trousseau, Armand, 85
Tumor cell proliferation, 22
Tumors, solid, 3, 15, 49, 58, 107, 128, 136, 186
Turmeric, 30
2CDA, 18–19
2-chlorodeoxyadenosine. *See* 2CDA.
Tyrosine kinase inhibitor, 136
Tyrosine, 126

U
University of Arizona, Tucson, 11

University of California, Davis, 90
University of California, Irvine, 5, 19, 20, 145, 223
Unniversity of California, Los Angeles, 84, 131
University of California, San Francisco, 193
University of Connecticut, Storrs, 67
University of Illinois College of Medicine, Block Center for Integrated Cancer Treatment, 32
University of Indiana, 90
University of Michigan, Department of Urology, 29
University of Montreal, 31
University of Southern California, 80
University of Toronto, 157
Urea cycle, 148
Uterine cancer, 29

V
VA Greater Los Angeles Healthcare System, 61
Vanguard Cancer Foundation, 108
Vascular endothelial growth factor, 111
VEGF, 104
Vemurafenib, 150
Vinblastine, 23–24, 104
Vinorelbine, 114–115, 177–179, 180–181
Viruses, 44–46, 151–152
Vitamin C, 27

supplementation, 78
Vitamin E, 77
VP-16, 58

W
Warburg, Otto, 111, 149
Weil, Andrew, 69
Weinstein, I. Bernard, 138
Weisenthal, Larry, 11–12, 15, 21,
    24, 36, 48, 49, 97, 100
Whipple procedure, 84
White blood cells, 9, 153
Williamson, Sharon, 113–116
Wilshire Oncology, 96
Wine, red, 74–76
Woodcock, Janet, 167

Wortmannin, 138
www.PatientResource.net, 55
Wyeth Pharmaceuticals, 147

X
Xeloda, 106, 144–145
Xenoestrogens, 154–155

Y
Yale University, 10
Yoga, 28, 73
Young, Zhuang Su, 49

Z
Zieve, Robert, 194–195
Zocor (Simvastatin), 78

About the Author

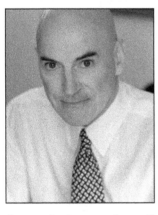

Robert A. Nagourney, MD, is the medical and laboratory director at Rational Therapeutics, Inc., in Long Beach, California. He is board certified in internal medicine, medical oncology, and hematology.

Dr. Nagourney received his undergraduate degree in chemistry from Boston University and his doctorate of medicine at McGill University in Montreal, where he was a University Scholar. After a residency in internal medicine at the University of California, Irvine, he went on to complete fellowship training in medical oncology at Georgetown University, as well as in hematology at the Scripps Institute in La Jolla.

During his medical oncology fellowship at Georgetown University, Dr. Nagourney confronted aggressive malignancies for which the standard therapies remained highly unsatisfactory. Responding to an unmet need, he pioneered the development of "personalized cancer therapy," applying a laboratory platform to match patients to therapies based on their unique response profiles.

As the founder of Rational Therapeutics, Dr. Nagourney has led in the development of "functional profiling" in human tumors.

Using human tumor microspheroids isolated directly from surgical specimens, this platform known as the Ex Vivo Analysis of Programmed Cell Death (EVA-PCD) measures drug-induced programmed cell death. The EVA-PCD has been shown to be a robust method for the prediction of clinical response to therapy.

With more than twenty years experience in this field, Dr. Nagourney has authored numerous manuscripts, book chapters, and abstracts. As a co-investigator on national cooperative trials, he introduced the use of platinum/gemcitabine doublets in the management of advanced ovarian and breast cancers, treatments that today are used around the world.

Dr. Nagourney resides in Long Beach, California, with his wife and two sons.

CPSIA information can be obtained
at www.ICGtesting.com
Printed in the USA
LVHW011916290921
699044LV00013B/507